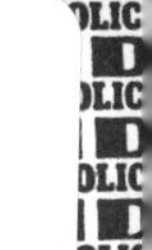

TOUCHING BOTTOM

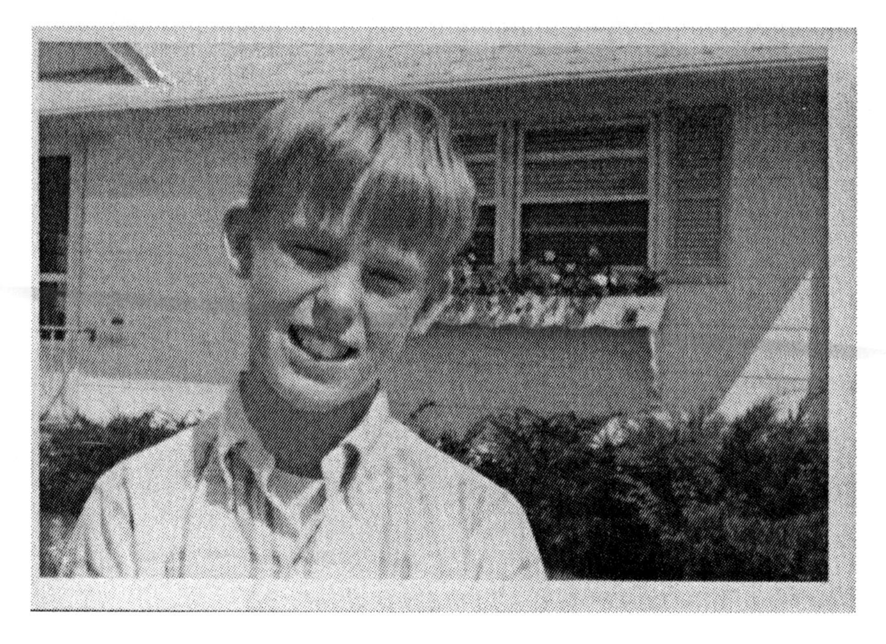

John, age 11.

To Georgine
Best Wishes,
[illegible]
a.k.a. Barbara Redmond

TOUCHING BOTTOM

A Story about Cancer, Death, and God's Love

BARBARA REDMOND

Writers Club Press
San Jose New York Lincoln Shanghai

TOUCHING BOTTOM

A Story about Cancer, Death, and God's Love

Writers Club Press
an imprint of iUniverse.com, Inc.

For information address:
iUniverse.com, Inc.
5220 S 16th, Ste. 200
Lincoln, NE 68512
www.iuniverse.com

ISBN: 0-595-19112-6

Printed in the United States of America

Epigraph

Loving-kindness and truth have met together;
Righteousness and peace have kissed each other.
Truth springs from the earth,
And righteousness looks down from heaven.

Ps. 85:10–11
New American Standard Bible

Contents

Preface

The following is an account of my own true story, written in the interests of cancer research. It is not a collection of medical data, for that is outside my realm of knowledge, but rather an account from the perspective of a cancer victim's parents. I do not know if it was simply a coincidence that I, the mother, was a freelance writer at the time. I only know that I took notes and vowed to write the story as soon as I knew the ending. But I found that I could not write it after the darkness of the storm. My sixteen-year-old son died.

Names and places have been changed to protect those less than innocent, for it is when the chips are down that emotions rise and souls are bared as great men grapple with the frightening aspects of the unknown.

***

A few years ago on *Good Morning America*, I saw an attractively dressed African-American woman in her forties tell the interviewer that her life was over. She was a member of Mothers Against Drunk Driving (MADD), a national organization. A drunken driver had killed her eighteen-year-old son, who was getting ready to go to college.

Not only had her own life ended, she maintained, but that of her entire family as well. She was saying, in effect, that they had all died when her son died. I wanted to reach out to her through the television screen and tell her not to grieve, to go on as if her son were still living. Based on my own experiences and what I learned after my son's death, I know that both of these young men are very much alive.

And so I write this story to help alleviate the suffering of this woman and others like her who have lost their dearest ones. Perhaps it will renew their hope.

ACKNOWLEDGEMENTS

To my children,
for their patience and understanding;

Beth, Howie, and Nadine,
for their loving support;

Frank, an editor, who
made me stretch a little further
in the early stages of this work; and

Rick, who edited the final draft
and advised me during the completion
of this project.

I also wish to thank Bill,
for his technical expertise;

Anita, who gave to me, a stranger,
her reading and editing skills;

Jill, Duke, Nancy, and Barbara
for their help and encouragement; and

Mary Alice, who read the final copy
and provided helpful input.

Because this book is an account
of a personal journey,
I feel particularly indebted to Mary Lou,
who never wavered in her belief in me
or the contents of this book.

Through her friendship, ideas, and feedback,
she encouraged me to bring this book to fruition.

Premonition

Intuition—a woman's hot line to God—is a built-in ambulance siren sounding an alarm to mothers when their children are in danger. It works for animals as well; a mother bear, for instance, protects her cubs from annihilation without instruction. However, a premonition, which is also an instinctive foreboding, differs from intuition in that it is an actual warning of something yet to occur.

I drove our station wagon along Route 20, an interstate highway that ran through the city, with sixteen-year-old Lynn in the passenger seat beside me. I had four children, but she was my only daughter. I was looking forward to shopping with her, but in 1970 our youths were rebelling against the Establishment, and teen-agers were rejecting most of the standards that their parents upheld. This made our outing something of an ordeal.

We were discussing where we would shop for Lynn's back-to-school clothes. When I suggested Pittman's, she rolled her eyes and said, "I'm not going there!"

I looked at her in wonderment. "What's wrong with Pittman's?" I asked. Pittman's was one of our city's two leading department stores.

"Because—they're awful—they're old-fashioned," she replied.

Lynn's taste in clothes had always differed from mine. I recalled visiting every possible store in Cobourg and the nearby mall to find her confirmation dress.

"Well, what about Bergman's then?" I proposed. Bergman's was a fashionable department store in Dickinson, twenty miles east.

"Bergman's!" she scoffed. "I'm not getting their ugly stuff!"

Dismayed, I slowed the car and glared at her. What was wrong with her today? I wanted our morning together to be fun.

"Well, where then?" I retorted. What was wrong with teen-agers anyway? Why couldn't we get along?

"The Army & Navy Store," she replied.

"The Army & Navy Store!" I echoed. What in heaven's name would it have that she'd want? I had shopped there before, but only once or twice to get special sports items for the boys.

Suddenly, I felt a powerful force grip the steering wheel, and we swerved. I braked to slow down, but feeling I'd lost control, I screamed, "Oh, my God, help me!" Steering the car onto the shoulder of the road, I managed to edge it along a four-foot embankment, where we sped along on the gravel some distance before we stopped.

Both of us sat silent, stunned, staring straight ahead. After a few minutes, I started to drive along, when suddenly a dark cloud came over me, an ominous presence surrounded me, and I had a foreboding that something terrible was going to happen to Lynn's younger brother, John. I glanced at Lynn, but she sat motionless, still staring straight ahead. Noticing her set jaw, I had the impression that she thought it was her choice of stores that had shocked me into swerving the car and braking quickly. Therefore, I drove on, saying nothing, with that scary incident locked in my memory.

***

John, the third of our four children, was easy to love right from the start. One can hardly help but love a good baby. Five years younger than his brother Rob and two-and-a-half years younger than Lynn, John was born on the Fourth of July. His birth upset our plans. Just the year before, we had purchased our first house, a two-bedroom ranch. Once John arrived, it was already too small for us.

Immediately, relatives attributed his looks to his namesake, my father, John, who had the same long and slim face, blue eyes, and lean body. Although John's blond hair differed from his grandfather's dark brown hair, my relatives reasoned that blond hair "ran in the family." My parents, both dark-haired, had produced six children, four with dark hair and two with blond.

From the beginning, John didn't seem to want to cause any trouble. Upon awakening from his afternoon nap, sleepy-eyed, he would lie or sit quietly in his crib and play with his toys. After school, Rob and Lynn entertained him in his crib until I was ready to pick him up and change him, and he rarely cried for me to do that.

Unlike the older children, John never needed to assert himself. From infancy until the time he went to school, he just tagged along with the crowd good-naturedly. We were always in a hurry. If we made plans to go on a picnic, we talked about it with Rob and Lynn, and then just grabbed John up and carried him out to the back seat of the car. Halfway there, we would tell him what we were going to do. Any plans we had made were all right with him.

Those pre-school years passed quickly, insignificantly, but John's second day of kindergarten will always be memorable. Rob and Lynn had already left on the school bus, and I drove John to the elementary school nearby. I accompanied him to his class on the first day to acquaint him with his new surroundings, but on the second day I sat in the car out front, watching and waiting for him to go in. He ran up the steps, then turned around and stood there for a minute, looking wistfully at me. Then, holding one elbow tight to his side, he raised his forearm and moved each finger singularly until he formed a shy wave. I waved back, but after he went inside, I swallowed hard as I drove away. What a major step that first day of independence is in one's lifetime!

The next few years flew by. My husband, Jack, owned and operated an electrical contracting business, and I managed the office from our home. Christopher was born when John was four, and so, along with the business, I had four children under the age of ten to care for.

Suddenly, John was twelve and in middle school. With our permission, he took over Rob's paper route. One year later, he had acquired enough money to buy skis and ski poles at Crown Point, a nearby resort. When he asked our permission to buy skis that fall, he pointed out that all of his friends skied at Crown Point, including Pat Douglas, his best friend, who lived next-door. In addition, his school provided both a bus to drive the youngsters to Crown Point once a week after school and a male teacher who served as a chaperone.

After some discussion, we agreed to let John participate in this activity. Skiing was a good, clean sport. High school students using drugs was beginning to be a problem now, and we were concerned about providing him with a healthy alternative.

***

Within weeks, the nightly frosts had turned the green leaves on the trees and bushes to harmonious reds, yellows, and golds. In the warm autumn sunshine, vineyard owners displayed their Concord grapes and hardy mums on roadside stands along the glistening lakes. Farmers set out their squash, Indian corn, gourds, apples, and pumpkins to sell. It was harvesttime.

Soon thereafter, shimmering snowflakes fell, with ten inches arriving in one night. John, Pat, and Tom Jackson, another neighbor boy who lived down in front of us, got out their ski gear and decided to test it on our hill.

After school one afternoon, I was making a dish of scalloped potatoes and ham for dinner. As I carried the casserole over to the oven, I glanced out the kitchen window and caught a glimpse of John's red wool hat flying past me down the hill. Curious, I paused to look further. Apparently he and his friends had fashioned from the hard-packed snow a ski jump that was about six feet high and only a few inches wider than the width of two skis. John was now crouched in a position to mount it.

I held my breath, watching. One misjudgment could send him sprawling. Since bindings could not be relied upon to release skis from ski boots at that time, skiers frequently broke their legs. I muttered,

"Oh, John!" At the bottom of the run, only a ditch separated him from the busy state road below.

As he trudged back up the hill carrying his skis, I yelled out the window. "John, don't go off that ski jump again! That's dangerous!"

John shrugged it off. "It's not dangerous, Mom. It's fun! Nothing will happen!"

The previous winter, John had begun to watch world-class skiers on television soaring like birds as they glided off ski jumps and landed upright. When I saw that he revered their grace and agility, I explained, "They practice for years, John, before they land that smoothly. They aren't able to do that when they first start skiing!" But John, smitten by his newly-discovered skills, turned a deaf ear. Certain factions in our society were undermining parental authority now, and the slogan for youths was "If it feels good, do it!"

"Oh, John. Please don't!" I repeated, and again that foreboding dark cloud encompassed me.

A few nights later, Jack, while finishing his after-dinner coffee, looked at the daring antics of the young skiers through the picture window of our dining room. The snow-covered hill was illuminated by floodlights on the back of our house, the house next door, and the two neighboring houses below us.

Jack had lettered in three sports—football, basketball, and baseball. Ignoring his doctor's orders, he had once played on the football team with a dislocated shoulder. His loyal teammates provided the cover so that his parents never knew about it. Although the shoulder still hurt when he lay on his right side in bed, he had no regrets about the price he had paid for that thrill.

"Jack, make John stop," I begged. "What he's doing is dangerous! He'll get hurt! I just know it!"

Thinking me overprotective, Jack replied, "He won't get hurt! All it takes is a little coordination!" Fully aware of my lack of agility, Jack thought that I could not comprehend inborn sports ability. We had been in school together from the fourth grade through high school, and we had shared many laughs over the numerous times I had bent my thumb back while trying to catch the softball in gym class.

So, that night, Jack insisted that I leave John alone. "Whatever he does, let him do it! If he gets hurt, it's worth it!"

"Oh, Jack!" I protested again, but I did not detail my reasons. Jack would have given no credence to my fearful premonition. Although he had deep religious convictions, he was also a realist. He scoffed at news accounts of UFO sightings and supernatural happenings that were being reported daily.

As I stood at the window that night and silently watched the reckless young skiers fly by, I wished that I, too, could dismiss the premonition as nonsense. But I realized that the powerful force I'd felt was stronger than I, and I could do nothing about it.

***

One day that February, a ski patrol volunteer telephoned us from Crown Point about 8:30 p.m. to say that John had had an accident. While skiing downhill, in order to avoid a collision with a young skier who had crossed in front of him, he had veered to the left and hit a tree stump. His leg hurt, but it was unlikely that it was broken. Could we meet them at the hospital about 9 p.m.?

At the emergency entrance, two volunteers slowly pulled John from the back of a Volkswagen bus. Although I said nothing, I was horrified to see that he was strapped to two boards nailed together like a cross. His body was upright, his arms were outstretched, and his legs were strapped to the vertical board.

Eyeing me sheepishly, John forced a laugh and said, "It doesn't hurt, Mom. Don't worry!"

All I could say was, "Oh, John," over and over again.

In the waiting room, the ski patrol volunteer stayed with us for three hours while John was in surgery. After two hours had passed, Dr. Ferreira, the orthopedic surgeon, came down to tell us that the X-rays showed a broken femur, the long bone extending from the pelvis to the knee. Taking us aside, he said in low tones that they would have to put John in traction.

"For how long?" we asked.

"Four weeks." Dr. Ferreira stared at the floor, not wanting to see the dismayed looks on our faces.

The next morning, before John went up to surgery, the doctor explained that they would have to put a pin in John's leg just below the knee to hold the leg in traction. During this three-hour procedure, I had plenty of time to meditate, and although John had ignored my concerns about taking risks on the ski jump, I knew in my heart that this time there would be no complaints. No, I would just be thankful that John's injury was only a broken leg that in time would heal.

After the surgery, John's skiing buddies and schoolmates swarmed around him admiringly. To them, he was a hero. He was flattered that they wanted to autograph his cast with colorful Magic Markers, and he pretended not to mind that he was bedridden—until one day when we were alone. After giving me a terrified glance, he rolled his eyes frantically. "Mom," he demanded, "how can I stand to be tied down like this for four weeks, to say nothing about the pain?"

"Just take it one day at a time, John," I said. "Every morning when you wake up, say to yourself, 'I'll just try to get through this day.' That's the best that you can do, honey!" Wide-eyed, he searched my face to see if I meant it. Finally, he said he guessed he'd try it.

So John endured each day by counting the remaining weeks, days, hours, and minutes until he would be well again. His friends came daily after school, laden with gifts such as hamburgers from Skip's, candy, and puzzles. Above his head, they suspended two round acrylic clinkers that were tied to opposite ends of a cord on the traction equipment. For a week, John, mesmerized by their harsh sound, clanked them together endlessly until the nurses, in order to preserve their sanity, took them away from him.

After crossing off the four weeks on the calendar one day at a time, John learned that, for enduring the pain and confinement in traction, his prize was a body cast extending from his armpits to his toes, with a broomstick handle plastered in between his legs to separate them.

As we took our son out the door to go home, Dr. Ferreira called after him, "Five weeks this time, John!" This news shocked all three of us, but John, smiling feebly, accepted it and did not complain.

Through the snows and winds of March and the budding greens of April, John endured five more weeks restrained in bed at home, with a choice of stretching out flat on his stomach, rolling onto his back, or lying on his side with one leg up in the air. He whiled away the days watching television, visiting with his skiing buddies after school, and studying with tutors in the evening. One or two girls also came after school to play Life or Monopoly with him.

Finally, with a new zest for living, John burst out of his plaster cocoon, and was able to walk on crutches. On Memorial Day, he went outside and waved a flag, emoting and letting the warm sun nourish his wilted body.

But later in June, my blood chilled as I looked out a bedroom window one day and saw him hobbling toward our neighbor's house to return the borrowed crutches. Instead of walking normally, as he was able to do, and carrying the crutches, he was using them! A lump rose in my throat, and I swallowed hard. *Why wasn't John rejecting the crutches? The doctor had told him that he could now walk without them.* Apprehension gripped me again. *Everything terrible that was going to happen to John had already happened, hadn't it?*

In July, Dr. Ferreira, satisfied that the bone had healed properly, discharged John with no restrictions. He was so thin and fragile, however, that I kept him in after school for a few weeks despite his insistence that he felt fine. Finally, I gave in and let him resume his paper route.

One day in August I drove past John as he was walking with a friend along the road near our house. He was carrying a full bag of newspapers on one shoulder, and it struck me that his spine curved noticeably. That night, I cautioned him, "Stand up straight, John. You're leaning to one side! Your leg is better now. There is no reason to walk lopsided anymore!"

"Yeah, yeah, I know," he said. But whenever I passed him walking down the road after that, he was still leaning to one side.

Every night, I would remind him again. "Stand up straight, John!"

"For Pete's sake, Mom, leave me alone!" he said. "I feel fine. I'm not sick. My leg doesn't hurt. Stop nagging!"

"Okay, John," I replied, but I was so concerned, I couldn't resist adding, "But you're not standing up straight!"

The hot summer days passed, and before school started, we decided to go to the ocean on a four-day vacation over Labor Day weekend. The night before we left, I assigned jobs for all four of the children to do, and when John did not finish his, I reprimanded him. "John, you don't have your chores done! How come? Are you getting lazy or what?" He had always been a good worker.

Unable to bear my scolding, he broke down. "My back hurts, Mom," he finally admitted. "I can't lie down at night. I have to get up and do exercises so I can go to sleep."

"It does? You do? Well, it's about time you told me, John. You're going back to Dr. Ferreira when we get home!"

However, when we returned from the ocean, John felt better, and I thought that perhaps he had just walked prematurely on the mended leg. "You should give up your paper route, John," I said. "Get someone else to do it. I think the papers are too heavy for your back to carry yet. I'm going to take you back to see Dr. Ferreira."

On the following Tuesday, when we walked into Dr. Ferreira's office, John, tanned from the seashore, looked the picture of health. He was limping only slightly and leaning a bit to one side.

When Dr. Ferreira came out of the examining room, he sat down behind his desk, and John and I sat opposite him. Narrowing his eyes sympathetically, he looked directly at John and said quietly, "You have a curvature of the spine, John."

Turning quickly to me, he added, "Look up your insurance to see if you're covered, and call me. Then bring him back for X-rays."

John and I were stunned. We drove home in silence, and on the way I prayed, "Please, dear God, what should we do about it?"

Two weeks later, when I called for an appointment with Dr. Ferreira, I learned that the doctor was out of town for two weeks. *Perhaps by the time he returned, John would be better.*

Time passed, but nothing changed. John still dragged his leg as he walked, and he leaned to one side. Otherwise, he felt good, except for a brief pain in his side at night.

When I finally did reach Dr. Ferreira on the phone, he asked anxiously, "How is he?"

"Well, he seems to feel better."

"Take him swimming," he said. "Exercise will be good for him." But when we went to an indoor pool, John, who had always been an avid swimmer, would only sit by the side of the pool, saying that swimming made him feel suffocated.

Each day I sought direction from Saint Jude, the patron saint of hopeless cases. He had helped me before through difficult times. I did not understand it, but I felt as if I were suspended in air, trying to escape a nameless, menacing plague hovering over me.

One evening John hobbled through our basement door with his best friend, Pat, following him. Coming over to me in the laundry room, where I was folding clothes, John looked up at me with twinkling blue eyes and said innocently, "Mom, I just fell off my bike and hit the road on the end of my spine!"

Looking down at him, I paled. "Oooh, John!" I exclaimed.

"No, Mom," he insisted, "it felt good. I could feel it tingling all the way up my spine!"

The next day, I was pleasantly surprised to see him walking down the stairs normally instead of haltingly. He had been coming down, one step at a time, favoring one leg.

It was now November and soon we would learn the real reason for John's leaning and limping. Only then would we realize that he was in a truly precarious position.

The Examination

That day, during an examination in his office, Dr. Ferreira suddenly looked up and exclaimed, "Oh, I know what it is!" Then, quietly, he said, "John may have a tumor!"

Jack paled, and I turned ashen. Seeing our reaction, he quickly reassured us, "Oh, it's nothing. It's probably benign. I'll call Dr. Hofmann at St. Luke's Hospital. Have you heard of him? He's a neurosurgeon. He does all of his work at St. Luke's. He's good." We had not heard of him. Fortunately, there had never been any serious illnesses in either of our families.

Nevertheless, the word *neurosurgeon* rang a bell with me. Only the week before, my brother Joe and I had talked about John's problem when we were visiting at my parents' house in Middletown. Joe, twenty years older than I, was a full professor at the State University of Riverside.

"I'm so worried about John's leg," I had told him. "The doctor says that he should swim to exercise it, but I don't know. John's posture has changed completely."

Three years before, Joe's twenty-eight-year-old son, Mike, had broken his leg while skiing. "It was two years before Mike's leg was back to normal," Joe had informed me. "He walked with a limp all the time. But there's one thing I know about doctors—I'd never let a neurosurgeon touch me!"

His words echoed in my ears that day in Dr. Ferreira's office—and again the next day when we met with the neurosurgeon at St. Luke's Hospital in Dickinson.

The weather was unpredictable that gray afternoon when we drove to the hospital—first raining, then snowing. Dr. Hofmann, a six-foot, dark-haired man of fifty wearing black, horn-rimmed glasses, came into our private room and closed the door behind him. Shaking hands with Jack and nodding to me pleasantly, he placed his black satchel at the foot of John's bed. After greeting John, he sat down on the bed beside him. Turning toward Jack, he asked, "How long has the boy been ill?" A native of Austria, he spoke with a German accent.

"About three months," Jack replied. "Since August."

"Why didn't you come then?" Dr. Hofmann inquired.

"Because we didn't know that anything was wrong," Jack answered. "He broke his leg last February. We thought it was a muscle weakness. He had no pain—only an ache in his side."

The doctor reached into his black bag and took out a tuning fork. Pulling back the white seersucker bedspread and the sheet below it, he ran the tuning fork over John's left hip and asked, "Can you feel this?"

"Yes," John said.

Moving the instrument down to the knee, Dr. Hofmann queried, "This?"

"Yes."

Then Dr. Hofmann moved to the ankle. "This?"

"No."

My heart pounded.

Dr. Hofmann repeated the jab. "You cannot feel this?"

"No," John repeated, his cyes fixed on the ceiling.

The doctor pulled a giant safety pin from his pocket and pricked the bottom of John's left foot. "Can you feel this?"

"Yes."

"This?" He pricked the bottom of the right foot.

"Yes."

Then, returning to the left ankle, Dr. Hofmann asked, "But not this?"

Still staring at the ceiling, John swallowed hard and nodded.

"Close your eyes," the doctor said. He pushed John's big toe on the left foot forward. "Which way is your toe pointing—up or down?"

John guessed, "Up?"

"Which way now?" Dr. Hofmann pulled it toward him.

John, uncertain, replied, "Down?"

Dr. Hofmann moved to the right foot. He pushed the big toe upward. "Which way is the big toe pointing?"

For more than an hour, the doctor moved over John's body, prodding him from the waist down.

Finally he put the tuning fork back into the black bag, placed the safety pin back inside his jacket pocket, and walked over to the window. Standing there with his back to us, he latched his thumbs in the armholes of his navy blue pinstriped vest and gazed outside at the falling snowflakes for several moments.

He then turned around and came over to my chair. For the first time, he addressed me. "The boy may have a tumor of the spine," he said slowly. Drawing his index finger across my shoulder blades, he added, "It may be right here." Chills ran through me.

Looking toward Jack, he continued, "We'll do a myelogram on Monday. We'll see then what we find." When Jack looked puzzled, he explained, "We do a lumbar puncture to introduce a substance opaque to X-ray into the spine so we can do an X-ray inspection of the spinal cord."

Jack did not reply. John lay still, listening.

After a brief pause, the doctor nodded and smiled at me. I, not wanting a final answer, said hopefully, "We'll just have to wait and see." Nodding again, Dr. Hofmann walked toward the door and paused there with his hand on the knob. Turning back to us, he said, "I wish you luck." My heart did not leap, however, because in his voice I sensed a tone of skepticism.

The next day, hospital aides moved John to a semiprivate room. The weekend passed uneventfully. Then came Monday morning.

***

When we arrived at the hospital to be with John for the myelogram, he was in good spirits. He had finished breakfast, sponge-bathed, and changed reluctantly from his blue block-print pajamas to the shapeless white hospital gown that tied at the neck and was open down the back. "Girl stuff," he grunted. His shoulder-length blond hair, disheveled now, was darkened with oily streaks from lack of shampooing.

John fiddled with the TV remote control that was clipped to the side of his bed and channel-surfed. It was a new toy to him; we did not yet have a remote control at home. He'd been given mild sedatives to calm him, and as noon approached, nurses gave him stronger medication before two aides slid him onto a gurney. Accompanied by a nurse, we followed them to a waiting room, where aides placed John in the corridor and departed.

He was lying with his head turned to one side. A white-haired nun in a street-length white habit came by. After checking John's identification band, she patted his head and whispered to us in the waiting room, "Is he yours?" When we nodded, her gray eyes lit up. Smiling, she said softly, "He's asleep." Patting his head once more, she went on down the hall. We would meet Sister Anastasia again. Her entire life revolved around this hospital.

Then all was quiet. The clock ticked away. Dr. Hofmann, taking long strides, walked past the door and turned left at the end of the hall, where he disappeared through a door. Soon a nurse came out that door and walked up the hall toward us. Looking at John's nametag, she called out his name to awaken him. Although groggy, he answered her, and with the help of another nurse, she wheeled him through the double doors. We then made our way to the waiting room.

***

A man came to the door and looked in, eyeing the television set on a shelf in the corner. About thirty-five, he wore olive-drab chino workman's pants and shirt and black shoes. One of his white socks had a hole that showed above the heel. Hands soiled with lubrication grease, he walked over to the TV, turned on the volume, and waited a minute. When a picture did not appear on the screen, he snapped the volume control off and on again. Reaching around behind the set, he jiggled the cords plugged into the wall outlet, then squatted down and peered under the set. Several times he snapped the volume control button on and off, but the screen remained blank.

"Damn it," he muttered.

He jerked the cords again and snapped the same controls but to no avail. Finally, after another "Damn it all," he left.

I exhaled and said a prayer. *"Thank you, God. Please, dear God, let him fix a television set somewhere else today."* I needed to be alone with my thoughts. *"Please God, let them find what you want them to find."* I was weary. It had taken so long to get this far.

As I glanced toward the opposite wall, I noticed a lifelike oil painting illuminated from above by a horizontal light encased in a gold frame. In the painting, a middle-aged man with thinning black hair streaked with gray at the temples appeared to be staring at me. A small gold plaque beneath the painting identified him as "Malcolm Bliss, Benefactor of St. Luke's Hospital." A faint smile showed at the corner of his lips. I felt his compassionate gray eyes upon me. He seemed to be saying, "Don't worry, dear. Everything will be all right."

Deliberately, I pulled away from his stare and glanced around quickly, embarrassed, hoping that no one had seen me mesmerized. Jack and I were alone in the room, and he was reading. I wondered then if that man was really looking at me. I decided I must have been dreaming.

Two hours may have passed. I can't be sure because time is timeless when one is praying. Jack left to get some coffee. When he came back, everything was the same, except that the chairs felt harder. I squirmed, crossed and uncrossed my legs, sat with one leg tucked up under me, and shifted from one buttock to the other. Finally, a nurse came out the door of the examining room and walked toward us.

"Mr. and Mrs. Redmond?"

"Yes," we replied in unison.

"The doctor will be right out. He wants to see you."

"Thank you," we muttered.

My arms and legs were numb from the long hours of sitting. I had smoked more than usual. Whatever the outcome was, I was eager to hear it. I just wanted to get it over with.

Finally, Dr. Hofmann, still in his green scrubs, strode down the hall. My eyes searched his face for an answer, but he gave no clue. Jack and I stood up and faced him, like two prisoners before a judge, waiting to hear the sentence.

"Mr. and Mrs. Redmond?"

"Yes," we replied.

"We've examined your son. We've determined a growth on the spine—probably a tumor. We'll operate tomorrow, if that's all right with you. I may have to remove some vertebrae."

"How many?" Jack asked.

"Probably four."

"How long will it take?"

"Four hours."

"Is it serious?"

"Yes, it's serious."

We nodded, understanding.

Then I reached out to Dr. Hofmann. "We'll be with you in our prayers tomorrow, doctor."

Looking down at the floor, he nodded. "All right."

"This growth could be benign?" I asked.

"Yes," he replied. Then, hesitating, he added, "But so often in children they are malignant."

Five years ago, Tony Schwartz wrote that, until the 1960s, everything was still in the closet. People didn't speak of homosexuality, battered wives, date rape, or sexual abuse. It was deemed inappropriate to talk about your personal feelings. Even the word *cancer* was not spoken in polite society.[1]

In the early 1970s, cancer was a silent menace and the most dreaded word in the English language. We stood there for a moment in silence. I reeled. "Dear God," I prayed, "am I dreaming? Is this a nightmare?" In anguish, I looked again, but this man in the green scrubs who stood before us was real.

After aides had returned John to his room, we left the hospital. At home that night, fighting tears, I swallowed hard, tightening up, choking back. But finally the tears came, like floodwater bursting over a dam—strong, gushing, continuous. How could I say that my world had ended? That I wanted to get off. That my life had become nothing but heartbreak? It was as if I were a dish heaved against the wall, shattered into a million pieces.

Finally the tears subsided. I picked up the kitchen phone and dialed an old friend, Father Burrell, who was a priest at St. Vincent's Church. When he answered, I sobbed, "Father Burrell, the most terrible thing has happened. My son has—a—tumor in the—spinal cord! He'll have—surgery—tomorrow." I could hardly get the words out. "Father—Burrell, will you—pray for him?"

"Of course I will, dear," he assured me. "I'll pray for him at Mass in the morning, and I'll pray for you, too. Now don't worry, dear. We'll storm the heavens with prayers." That evening, the three priests at St. Vincent's devoted their entire supper hour to prayers for us in our crisis.

I hung up the phone, then lifted the receiver and dialed again. This time I called my mother, a widow, who lived 150 miles north of us in Middletown. Since she was forty years old when I was born, she was eighty-six now. I was the youngest of her six children. Although she was still physically active, her mind sometimes failed her. When she answered

---

[1] Tony Schwartz, *What Really Matters*, New York: Bantam Books, 1995.

the phone, I started to cry. Finally, I blurted out, "Mom, I have—the worst—news. I can—hardly—tell you."

"Why, Barbara, what is it?" she pressed me.

"It's John." Sobbing, I told her the story.

"Will you pray for him?" I begged.

"Oh, Barbara, that's dreadful," she replied. "John's such a nice little boy. The priest is coming in the morning to bring me communion. I'll ask him to pray for John, and I'll pray too."

Next, I telephoned our pastor. "Father Brennan? It's John—operation—tomorrow. Will—you—pray—for him—at Mass tomorrow?"

"Yes, yes, of course I will, dear," he replied. Then he asked, "Who will do the operating?"

"Dr. Hofmann," I answered.

"He's a good man," the priest said in sober tones. "He's the best in this area of the state, and from what I hear, he's very dedicated." This was heartening news. We knew so little about the man who held the fate of our son in his hands.

Hanging up the phone, I walked over to the cupboard where I kept the medicine. I pulled out a bottle of pills that I had purchased the day before on the way to the hospital. The label read, "500 mg. Aspirin, Time-Released." Because I never took medicine—only vitamins—I considered it daring to take 1,000 milligrams of aspirin, but I knew that I must. With a glass of water, I swallowed two pills to help me through the night. Although I would sleep the sleep of the damned, I would awaken with new hope in the morning.

***

That same evening, while I was crying at home, Jack went back to the hospital. Finding John asleep, he sat in a chair by his bed, keeping vigil. About 8 p.m., a man dressed in a business suit came in and walked over to the bed, calling out loudly, "John Redmond? John Redmond?"

John stirred, barely answering.

Jack, feeling edgy, stood up and snapped, "Hey, watch what you're doing! Can't you see he's asleep?"

"Oh, that's right, I guess he was," the man answered. "Well, anyway, John, I'm Dr. Lawson, and I'll be giving you your anesthetic tomorrow." Jack pulled back, surprised. He had not expected to see a doctor dressed in street clothes.

Hardly opening his eyes, John nodded slightly. "Oh, OK." Silently, Dr. Lawson copied some data from the chart at the foot of the bed and left.

Then Dr. Hofmann came in. John, awake now, was listening. Unconvinced of the diagnosis, Jack first asked Dr. Hofmann about the lump that had appeared on the myelogram. Was he positive that it was a tumor?

"No," Dr. Hofmann answered. "It could be a blood clot."

Jack persisted. "What will happen if you take four vertebrae out? He's a good baseball player right now—in fact, a pitcher." John had played baseball, football, basketball, and hockey since he was nine years old.

"Well, he certainly won't be able to participate in sports," the doctor replied.

"What will happen if you don't operate?"

"He'll be paralyzed from above the waist down."

John lay frozen in silence.

Dr. Hofmann, ready to leave, assured Jack that he would have the nurses check John every hour throughout the night. If there was danger of imminent paralysis, he would operate at any hour. Otherwise, the surgery would be at 1 p.m. the next day, as scheduled. As the doctor went out the door, Jack followed him.

John called after him, "Dad, are you leaving?"

Jack had momentarily forgotten John. "Yes, John, I think I'll go home. You try to get some sleep. We'll see you in the morning."

"Dad?"

"Yes, John?"

"Oh, nothing...." But after a pause, he repeated, "Dad?"

"Yes, John?"

"Nothing. Turn out the light as you leave. It shines in my eyes. Yes, I'll see you in the morning."

***

We headed for the hospital early, down the snow-speckled turnpike to Dickinson. That morning, I told John something that I later regretted, afraid that I might have destroyed his faith.

Aware of the possible consequences of the surgery, he was now crippled with fear, and he had stopped asking questions. From the confident Little League pitcher who carried the game, he had reverted to the miserable child with chicken pox whom I'd rocked in my arms and comforted. With his brow drawn into a frown, he kept one eye closed and the other half-open, on me. Even though he was sedated—half-awake, half-asleep—he couldn't hide his anxiety.

For consolation, I sat beside him, patting his arm, and the deep lines in his forehead lifted. In my heart, I wanted to tell him something that I believed would give him strength to go up for surgery. But knowing how he questioned the validity of religion, I wondered if I dared. At that time liberal clergymen were encouraging young people to reject the traditional beliefs of their parents. Nonetheless, I wanted to help my son. Mustering up my courage, I started, "John?"

"Mmm-hmm." Eyes closed now, he stirred a little.

"John, you know if you believe that He'll help you, He will."

Certainly God in his mercy and kindness and love would answer a prayer from a boy who asked only to walk.

His eyes opening now, he nodded his head. "I know—I am," he said plaintively.

When I returned from the cafeteria after lunch, Dr. Hofmann was in John's room, checking his charts. He was standing with his back to me. I suddenly felt an urgent need to talk with this man again who dared to work on backs. I had to let him know that today he would be working on a very special back, one that differed from any back he had ever seen before. This back belonged to my own flesh and blood. Impulsively, I walked up behind the doctor and put my hands around his waist.

"Dr. Hofmann?" I began.

He wheeled around, surprised.

Motioning toward John, I continued, "You're going to do a good job up there today. Everything's going to be all right." Upon awakening that morning, I had felt more positive, less burdened. It must have been the prayers.

"All right," he smiled, good-naturedly.

I hesitated, then added, "And Dr. Hofmann…."

"Yes?"

"I just want you to know that we'll be with all of you in our prayers, every step of the way."

"All right," he said again, seriously. Then, looking over at John, he conjectured, "Maybe it's only a blood clot."

I left to get a drink of water. When I returned, the doctor was just coming out of the room. As we passed each other in the corridor, he searched my eyes intensely. I looked back at him confidently.

When the orderlies came to take John to surgery, I rose from the chair by his bed and looked down at his half-glazed eyes and his tousled blond hair. They slid him onto the gurney and led the way to the elevator, motioning for Jack and me to follow. When they opened the elevator door on the fourth floor, I saw a door directly across the hall from us marked, "SURGERY—KEEP OUT." The aides pushed John out into the hall and stepped aside so that we could have a moment alone with him.

We made light of it, laughing, and said, "Well, so long, kid. We'll see you later!" I reached for his hand and squeezed it. But as I started to leave, he gasped and rolled his eyes backward toward me, as if he were drowning. I bent over close to his face and whispered, "Pray, John!"

Swinging back the double doors, they wheeled him into the surgery. The doors closed behind them. John now had to face it alone. We could not be there with him.

Nurses directed us to the waiting room on the main floor, where we were to stay until after the surgery. When Jack left to get a cup of coffee, I saw Dr. Hofmann outside in the hall, waiting to take the elevator up to surgery. Spotting me, he waved and called out kindly, "I'll call down so you won't have to worry."

Zero Hour

But the phone didn't ring. For five hours, I prayed, "Hail Mary, full of grace; please be with them."

During that fifth hour, Jack was uneasy. He left to go to the cafeteria for dinner. Because I did not feel like eating solid food, he offered to bring me some Jell-O. Soon thereafter, a young woman came in from a nearby desk and said that they had just called down from surgery. Our son had a tumor. The doctor would be down shortly.

"Did they say what kind?" I asked.

"No, they didn't say," she replied, exiting quickly.

Fifteen minutes passed before the doctor, in his green scrubs, stepped off the elevator. He came over to me where I was sitting alone in the waiting room. He sat down beside me and reached for my hand.

"It was a tumor," he started.

I listened carefully. I had trouble understanding his German accent.

"It was?" I replied faintly.

"I took out the back part of four vertebrae." Using one hand, he spread his thumb and little finger seven or eight inches apart. "That much," he said. I thought it strange how he measured distance. I had always seen it measured with both hands, using the two index fingers.

I attempted to ask the terrible question. "Was it…?" But I couldn't finish.

"Yes," he said quietly. "It was malignant, and there's more in the spinal cord."

"There is!"

"We can't touch that," he explained in a low voice.

"I understand."

"But I called Dr. Morello from the Benjamin Taylor. He was interested and came right over. He does a new kind of surgery for this type of tumor. It's very exacting work. It has to be done with a microscope, and he's up there now working on it. I'll go up and do another operation and come back and close your son up later.

"I'm sorry," he added quietly. After a moment, he started to pull his hand away. I immediately reached out and grabbed it and put it back on mine. I felt as if I were drowning, and his hand exuded such strength. Yet I felt ashamed that I had to lean on him. He had just spent five hours with my son in surgery.

My eyes fell to the floor. I managed to ask, "Dr. Hofmann, do you believe in prayer?"

"Yes," he replied. I looked up to search his eyes, but he glanced away. My eyes went down again. I could not tell if he was merely accommodating me or if he meant it. But I sensed his defeat, and I felt driven to tell him, "Dr. Hofmann, you have divine guidance up there, you know."

"Yes, I know," he said softly.

Then, thinking of another time and another place, I inquired, "Dr. Hofmann, are you sure it's malignant? I know of a doctor who swore right after surgery that the patient's tumor was malignant, but when the biopsy came back, it was benign."

He shook his head. "No, it's malignant." Then, standing up, he said, "I've got to get back upstairs."

Just then, Jack walked up to us, carrying a dish of shaky red fruited Jell-O. "Dr. Hofmann has bad news for us, Jack," I said faintly, not looking at him. "It was a tumor. It was malignant."

"Yeah?" Jack answered, suppressing his shock. He asked the doctor, "How will the removal of the vertebrae affect him?"

Dr. Hofmann was quiet. Staring at the floor, he shook his head, as if to imply that that was the least of our worries.

By now, it was 6 p.m., and the buzz of young mothers, middle-aged men, old women, and grandfathers caring for young children filled the waiting room. Each carried a sorrow that only he or she fully understood. The same young woman from the desk came over again. With misty eyes, she offered to take us to a place where it was quiet. Thankful, we followed her to the elevator, where she directed us to the waiting room near the intensive care and surgery units on the fourth floor.

We found the small room, two sides of which were enclosed with half-walls of glass blocks. An attractive dark-haired woman about forty years old sat alone on the beige and green plastic-covered contemporary sectional. Copies of *U.S. News and World Report* and *Life* were strewn next to a black leather-bound Bible on the coffee table. The woman did not appear to be listening to the television in the corner, so I asked her if it would be all right to turn it off. She nodded.

Slouching in the corner seat beside her, I put my legs up on the coffee table and crossed them. Jack sat in a chair on the adjoining wall next to me. We lit cigarettes and stared into space, trying to digest our news. Please, God, I petitioned, do something. I wondered then about the bad impression it might make on the doctors if they came out of surgery and saw me, the mother of a cancer patient, smoking, after they had been in surgery slaving over my son, trying to save him.

Smoking was not banned in public places at that time. In 1966, on the recommendation of the Surgeon General, cigarette manufacturers were required for the first time to mark each pack with a label that warned of possible health risks, but smokers paid little attention. Health studies were being reported in the news media frequently, but since the findings were not consistent, the average person did not know what to believe.

I had always been a "social smoker." I smoked at morning gatherings of mothers with young children, or in the evening, after dinner, I had a few cigarettes with Jack over a cup of coffee. The practice of smoking was not generally frowned upon in society. On the contrary, it was considered fashionable in most circles. Yet here, in the hospital, I felt guilty about it.

But somehow I couldn't help myself. Smoking had become a nervous habit that seemed to soothe my nerves whenever I was faced with conflict or worry—and that was almost daily now.

Death Announcement on the Fourth Floor

In retrospect, it all seems hazy. As I recall, Dr. Hofmann, still in his green scrubs, and Dr. Morello came into the waiting room about 7 p.m. The doctors looked shocked when they saw me sprawled, half-sitting, half-lying, with my feet up on the table. I scrambled to straighten myself while Dr. Hofmann made the introductions. Dr. Morello, who was in his early fifties, was meticulously dressed in a brown double-breasted suit that accentuated his tall, lean frame. He had thinning dark hair and rimless glasses. A gold cap on his right front tooth shone as he greeted us.

"Dr. Morello is your new doctor," Dr. Hofmann said. "Your son is his patient now."

Looking up anxiously, I replied, "He is?"

Changing doctors had always made me feel insecure, and we had just gotten to know Dr. Hofmann. In the past, I had joked many times that John was born early just because I didn't want to change doctors. Dr. O'Bryan, my general practitioner, had booked a trip to Ireland just before my due date, and he had planned to turn me over to another doctor for the delivery. Although all of my other children were born two weeks late, John entered this world thirteen days early—on the Fourth of July—just two days before my doctor left for Ireland.

However, we couldn't complain too much in front of Dr. Morello about changing doctors. He had performed the microscopic surgery, and it would follow that he would carry the case through to completion.

"It's very bad," Dr. Hofmann said. "Dr. Morello agrees with me."

Pause. Dead silence. Finally, Jack asked, "How bad?"

"No hope—alive or dead." Dr. Hofmann glanced toward me.

"Really?" I said. He might as well have told me that they had just pushed a button to destroy the world. It didn't seem feasible. Whenever I had been in trouble, God had always come through for me. *Why, oh why, my God, have you abandoned me?*

"It must be God's will," I said. "He must want it this way." I knew that we must always pray for God's will, not ours, to be done. Only God, in his infinite wisdom, knows what our future holds.

The room was quiet. Nothing can really kill John, I thought. "I believe in life after death," I added. "John will live again." My voice trailed off. In a moment, my thoughts returned to the doctor. "What is the other alternative?"

"At the most, life in a wheelchair—paralysis from above the waist down."

"But John wouldn't like that," I countered. "I know him. He'd rather be dead!" In my mind's eye, I saw his legs, with Mercurochrome-covered scratches, dangling from a tree limb, with his body hanging upside down. I saw the tanned, skinny legs cavorting on the beach, then sprawling in the sand. I saw the blue-jeaned legs loping down the hill like the legs of a young colt broken loose from its mother. I saw the lean legs stretch and the muscles flex as he stood up, pumping the bicycle pedals.

"No, John wouldn't like that," I repeated. I lit another cigarette, and as I exhaled, I noticed that the room was filled with blue smoke. *A fine thing for the mother of a cancer patient,* I thought. But at that point, I felt compelled to smoke, although I knew that most doctors hated it. Just a few months before, during an office visit, a doctor had asked me to put out my cigarette.

My thoughts returned to the room. "Who will tell him?" I asked. "How can you tell a boy of thirteen that he's washed up—through? We know this boy."

Dr. Morello stepped forward. "We're not exactly heartless," he said. "We'll tell him for you."

"But he's only thirteen," I argued. "Why do we have to tell him?" The boy had a broken body. Did we also have the right to break him psychologically?

"Thirteen?" Dr. Morello scoffed. "Why, he's a man...."

A deathly silence permeated the room as each of us searched inwardly. Could we, even at our age, accept such news? Could we face being told of our imminent death, a death so terrible that even doctors and nurses withdrew from it in despair? Could any of us face life in a wheelchair? Would we simply melt away—kill ourselves? Or would we pray to God that it was not true, that we would wake up and find it had been just a horrendous nightmare?

"We may not have to tell him," Dr. Morello ventured finally. "Sometimes they don't ask. Sometimes they're afraid of the truth."

The words haunted me.

"Maybe he'll die," I said, hoping out loud. Looking up at the doctors, I added, "If he really is going to die, leave him alone. He's had enough." I thought of the four weeks he'd been in traction, the five weeks he had lain stiff in the body cast, the three months he'd been out of school, the anxiety again from summer into late fall, the X-rays, the myelogram, the worry before five hours of surgery, and the four vertebrae that had been removed.

"If God wants it this way, it's more humane not to fight it," I insisted. The doctors, still standing in the doorway, nodded in agreement.

I withdrew, staring at the floor as if drunk or dazed from a blow on the head. Presently, a hand touched my shoulder. It lingered there for a moment, and I heard a man say, "It will be hard on you." I did not look up. I was only aware that, after that, the man left the room. Having lapsed into a semiconscious state, completely obsessed with thoughts of John, I did not care who it was at the time. I suppose it must have been Dr. Hofmann.

Suddenly, I became aware that Jack and the woman sitting next to me had their eyes fixed on me, and it struck me that I should be crying. Normally, I would have cried at a time such as this. But I couldn't cry. I had prayed too long. I had read somewhere that the Jesus People said that they got high on Christ instead of drugs. I knew then that this was true because I had gotten high on Jesus that night. It had somehow allowed me to rise above my horrible circumstances—at least in part.

I stood up and reeled, muttering, "Well, I'm sorry. I'm numb." Seeking to remove myself from the situation, I made my way to the door and out into the hall. There I saw Dr. Hofmann standing with his back to the wall. Walking over to him, I said, "Dr. Hofmann?"

But when I looked up into his eyes, I saw a look of exhaustion and defeat—the look of a man who'd had enough of battling this eerie, elusive, gruesome foe that always seemed to come out on top.

"Dr. Hofmann, I'm not going to say too much. I know it's hard on you." I didn't want to burden him. He'd been in surgery six hours. "But Dr. Hofmann, I can't cry," I apologized. "I went home last night and cried it all out, and this morning I got up and just felt everything would be all right."

He nodded.

Then the words came back to me: *Maybe we won't have to tell him.*

"Dr. Hofmann, is there no hope—no hope at all—one way or another?" I had to have something to pray for.

He shook his head. It occurred to me that parents had pleaded with him before.

I stepped back. "Dr. Hofmann, there's just one more thing I want to ask you. John was in a skiing accident this year. When he veered to the left to avoid colliding with another boy who skied across the hill in front of him, he plowed into a tree stump and broke his femur. He was in traction and a body cast for nine weeks. Could the accident have caused this tumor? His father and I had this terrible argument about John skiing recklessly. I had a premonition about it, but his father overruled me. You see, his father loves sports."

"No," the doctor replied. "Malignant tumors are caused by the breakdown of cells." He never used the word *cancer*. "Sometimes, though, they'll form after an accident. I operated on a man not long ago who had a brain tumor, and he'd been in a car accident."

"Well, I'm glad to know that," I answered. Even though I would never blame Jack—he meant well—I had to know if my fears regarding that premonition were valid. My thoughts returned to John. "Dr. Hofmann, he'd have nothing to look forward to in a wheelchair, would he?"

He didn't say a word, but his eyes moved quickly from side to side.

"He'd be better off dead, wouldn't he?" I added, suddenly remembering all the promises God has made to us if only we keep His word—unimaginable joys in heaven, reunion with our loved ones, and happiness forever.

But I knew that the parting would be painful. "I'll see him again when I di—." I could not utter that terrible word. Shrinking away from the doctor, I wheeled around blindly, and landed in the arms of Sister Anastasia, who had been standing behind me, listening.

"You know that, don't you, Sister?" I cried.

Although we had met only once, we embraced each other. Tears rolled down her cheeks as she patted my back, comforting me. "Of course I do, child."

"Oh, Sister," I blurted. "I didn't mean to make you cry."

In that moment, she was the mother who had never hugged me, and I was the daughter she had sacrificed to devote her life to Him.

Then the three of us deliberated about whether John should live or die. Finally, Dr. Hofmann said, "It won't be up to us to decide," and suddenly a load lifted from my shoulders. I wondered then who would want the awesome burden of deciding for or against euthanasia, which was just then being introduced into our society. Who, other than God, could gaze into the crystal ball and see what the future held for another individual?

Suddenly a shrill female voice called over the loudspeaker, "Dr. Hofmann! Dr. Hofmann! Dr. Hofmann wanted in intensive care!"

Dr. Hofmann headed down the hall, and Sister Anastasia and I went back to the waiting room, our arms still around each other. Several moments later, the doctor looked in and called out to me, "That was your husband. He wanted to know about the skiing accident." With a nod of his head, he confirmed that they had discussed tumors and accidents.

Then Jack, who had followed Dr. Hofmann from intensive care, stuck his head in the door to ask if I wanted to see the doctor before he left.

"No." I said, looking up absent-mindedly. "No, I've been all over him." Suddenly realizing the ambiguity of my statement, we all laughed unrestrainedly. How strange it was that we could react like this, even when death was imminent.

"Would you like some grapefruit juice?" Sister Anastasia inquired.

It was 9 p.m. I had not eaten, and my adrenal glands had been working overtime. "Yes, I would. That sounds good," I said. As I drank the tangy beverage, I thought that it was the best I'd ever tasted. "Mmm. That's good," I said, gulping it quickly.

"Would you like some more?"

"Yes, I would. It was so good," I replied, handing her the empty glass.

Just then, Father Cyril, the hospital's chaplain, came in, and we started talking again about this terrible thing that had happened to my son. I started to cry, and I could not stop. "I'm sorry," I sniffed through a Kleenex. "I have my good and bad moments." Then I told them how I'd gotten through the morning on the prayers of the three priests and my mother. Prayers helped lift my burden.

"Would you like to have your son receive the Sacrament of the Sick?" Father Cyril offered.

"Oh, yes, I would."

"Would you like to have your son anointed?"

"Oh, yes, I would," I repeated.

He stood up and came over to the divan where I was sitting. "I'll give you the mother's blessing," he said, as he made the sign of the cross over my head. I had never heard of the mother's blessing. Then he went in to anoint John.

I started sobbing again. I had been unaware of the woman who was sitting next to me on the couch. Suddenly, she said, "You know, you don't want to give up hope. Only last week the doctors told me that my husband would never use his arms or legs again, but today they say he will.

He had a virus in the spinal cord. For some reason, the virus has mysteriously disappeared. That was only four days ago, so you see, you mustn't give up hope yet."

"Is that right?" I asked.

"A lot can happen in a few days," she continued.

When Father Cyril came back and Sister Anastasia returned from the kitchen, we talked about malignant cancer. "I had it," Sister Anastasia said. "On the side of my chin—where my habit rubbed. A doctor who never made eye contact with anybody noticed it. He said, 'What have you got on your face?'"

"That was it, all right," she went on, "but I've never had any trouble since." After reflecting on it for a moment, she shrugged her shoulders.

"Well, look at Father Tim from our monastery," Father Cyril interjected. "His malignant liver cancer had metastasized. The doctors couldn't touch it. He should have died, but he didn't. The cancer disappeared, and he's all right now. No sir, by gosh, we prayed for him like we never prayed before. We weren't going to let him go. He was a good man, and we needed him."

I mulled it over. Terminal cancer. I thought you always died from it eventually—that's what the term implied.

Sister Anastasia asked, "Would you like to have prayers said for your son?"

"Yes, I would," I replied.

"I'm going to call Mother Theresa over at the Benedictine monastery. Do you know where it is?" I shook my head. "The sisters pray there right around the clock," she explained. "I'm going to give them your son's name. I have great faith in them."

I knew the power of prayer, but this seemed like an imposition. I did not even know them. I reconsidered, however, thinking that perhaps the prayers would help alleviate the suffering for all of us. "Oh, thank you, Sister," I said.

Then Father Cyril inquired, "Would you like me to call our monastery down in South Hampton and ask them to pray for him?"

"I would," I said.

They left the room together, but Sister Anastasia came back to say that John's name was now on the sisters' prayer list at the monastery. "Would you like me to call Brother Bernard over at Mount Savior Monastery and ask them to pray for him?"

"All right," I answered.

After they had made the telephone calls, we sat and talked about the state of affairs in the world. The conversation turned finally to priests and vocations.

My spirits rallied. "I never realized until tonight," I said, "what a strength priests are." On reflection, I think Father Cyril was praying for us while we were there in his company.

"Yes," he agreed. "And it saddens me to see so many of our priests today cut down the laity, whom they're supposed to serve."

"Yes, I know what you mean," I answered. "I think it's too bad that priests don't pray for vocations. We need good priests."

"Pray for vocations?" He shook his head. "You just can't pray for some young person to serve God. That isn't right. Besides, I wouldn't pray for anyone to be a priest today." He grimaced. "It isn't easy."

"Nor is it easy to be anything else these days," I replied. "But we should pray that young people would seek out vocations, God willing. Not all young people should, or could, but we should pray that some *would.* I thought about how strange it was that I, the layperson, was sermonizing to the priest, instead of the other way around.

That night I dedicated my son to God, to serve Him in any way He wished, if only He would heal him.

After Surgery

As I walked down the corridors at St. Luke's the next day, the whole hospital seemed deserted. On my way to the intensive care unit, I asked God to give me the strength to face John. But when I saw him, he did not fit the image of a boy who was dying. He was rosy-cheeked, and he looked healthy.

As I entered the room, he was lying on his side. The nurse explained that she turned him every hour.

"Mom," he greeted me weakly. "Feel my right foot."

Apprehensively, I looked under the sheet and saw that he was wearing white surgical stockings. I took hold of his toes and pressed them together gently.

"Can you feel that, John?"

With eyes shut, he sighed, "Mmm-hmm."

"Now feel my left," he urged me.

I reached for the left foot and squeezed it.

"Can you feel that?"

"Mmm-hmm."

Going back to the right leg, I squeezed the flesh between his knee and his thigh. "Can you feel that, John?"

"Where are you?" he asked.

"On your right leg. Can you move it?"

He tried to flex the muscle, but nothing happened. He could only wiggle the toes a little.

"Not really," he said. "Try the left leg."

I repeated the procedure, pressing gently. "Can you feel that?"

"Mmm-hmm."

"Can you move it?"

Flexing the muscles, he drew the leg up perhaps two inches. A faint smile flickered across his lips.

"Good boy!" I said, my spirits rising. Turning to the nurse, a gentle, dark-haired woman in her early twenties, I said in a halting voice, "You know, this John—he's quite a fighter...." But a lump came up in my throat. I choked on the words and could not finish.

John nodded his head, his eyes lighting up in agreement.

How could you tell a boy like this that he was dying? The administration allowed both parents and visitors only five minutes in intensive care, but even that was too long. I turned my face away from John and said, "I'm going to get a drink. I'm thirsty." Hurrying out the door, I covered my face with my hands and fled down the hall past the nurses.

***

Larry L. King has written that "in the late 1960s...by their campus and street rebellions our kids made it clear that we [the parents] had not...[following World War II] attained our little slice of paradise to pass on to grateful heirs.... Their battle cry—'Don't Trust Anyone Over 30!'—implied that many of us had been failures. We were shocked and hurt...."

King referred to us as an "eager generation: ambitious to rise, intent on giving our children more than we had inherited of material things, dedicated to providing childhoods more of fun than of shadows.... Our generation learned early on that there was no free lunch, that precious little comes gift-wrapped.... We had worked so hard and come so far that many of us were blind to what was essentially a spiritual deficiency.... We didn't see that what we were offering them was materialism."

In contrast to our generation's fears about where our next meal would come from, and whether or not our parents could afford to buy us new shoes, he pointed out that our children feared atomic attacks in the Cold War, the violence of Vietnam, and the bloody Civil Rights wars in their own country that appeared right in front of them on television. "Our offspring may have stared into the terrible dark, wondering if their world literally might soon blow up," he noted.[2]

Rob and Lynn were a reflection of the times. Rob was a freshman at the local community college. Like his peers, he favored straight, shoulder-length hair, long sideburns, plaid flannel shirts, faded and torn blue denim jeans, and brown leather Western boots. Through their dress code, these students were sending a message that they were not concerned about materialism.

At first, we parents did not realize that our teen-agers and college students were playing a game with their elders. It could have been called "Shock the Establishment." Vying for position around the dinner table, first Rob introduced a controversial topic, then Lynn, a high-school sophomore, joined in. "What is wrong with drugs?" they would ask. Then they supplied their own answer: "No different than liquor."

"What is wrong with communism? Capitalism is synonymous with hoarding."

"What is wrong with communes? They share the work there."

"The Bible is a myth, isn't it?" Some of their teachers had told them that the Bible was "just songs of the poets."

Secularism had replaced religion. Young people asked questions but relied upon their own answers.

Trying to defend our values, Jack and I often overreacted. Dinner invariably resulted in indigestion. Tempers flared, verbal bullets flew, and the generation gap widened. At last, seeing the futility of seeking a resolution, we called a halt to these discussions, saying, "We have told you how we feel. Take it from there."

A strong bond had developed between the four of them. I had encouraged it because I wanted them to have the camaraderie and love that I'd never experienced with my siblings in my youth. We used humor in our

---

[2] Larry L. King, "Hey, Listen Up!," *Parade Magazine,* March 12, 1995, page 3.

conversations to teach them to laugh at themselves—even if it hurt. But John's illness separated them. Keen-witted Rob, stretched out on the family room floor watching television, was quiet now. Lynn lay in bed with a pillow over her head. Christopher went upstairs to be alone in the bedroom that he had once shared with John. As parents, we did not have the strength to console them. Like passengers on a wrecked ship, we drifted in all directions.

***

The third night after John's surgery, we came together as a family for dinner. Seated around the oval maple table in the dining room, we began to eat. But soon, appearing to choke on the food, our children pushed back their chairs, rose from the table, and scattered to leave the room through different exits. I stared straight ahead, dismayed to see them so grief-stricken.

Suddenly, I called out, "Come back, come back, all of you." Slowly, one by one, they filed back to their seats at the table.

Although we habitually took them to church on Sunday, we seldom discussed religion. It caused too much friction between us. However, in this difficult moment, something gave me the courage to speak up.

Looking at each of them around the table, I said, "You know, it's written in the Bible that Christ said, 'If two of you here on earth agree to ask for anything, my Father in heaven will certainly do it for you. For where two or three have come together to be with Me, there I am among them.'[3] As a group, let us ask for that help now."

Slowly, with hands in their laps, they lowered their heads and joined in as Jack began to recite the rosary. When we had finished, we ate and then rose from the table, each of us renewed with hope and the strength to continue.

***

---

[3] Matt. 18:19–20.

In the past, Rob had spurred John to glorious pitching triumphs for his Little League team. When he came into the kitchen at night, rushing past me toward the family room, he would ask, "How'd the kid do today?" Finding his brother, he'd repeat, "How'd you do, today, John? You struck 'em all out? Attaway to go, John. Keep your ball right over the center, and put it in there fast. Surprise 'em. That's what counts." As Rob talked, I had the impression that John was actually growing inches taller.

Rob took the news about his brother hard, although he was careful not to show it. One night at the hospital, however, when Jack took him out into the corridor and told him that John might never walk again, he began to cry, and he hit the wall with his fist.

The next night Rob asked me if he could buy an Irish setter from a college professor for $45, assuring me in the same breath that he had the money to pay for it. He worked part-time as a dishwasher at the Airport Restaurant to earn spending money.

Overwhelmed with problems, I put him off. "Oh, Rob, not now."

"The kid would like him," he urged. But I did not answer.

About 10 p.m. the next day, Jack and I arrived home from the hospital to find Rob and Beth, his college friend, standing in the dining room. Shawn was on a leash between them. The friendly dog, shivering with excitement at the sight of us, leaped up, wagged his tail, and pulled on his leash, trying to get closer.

Beth was in her bare feet, having left her snowy boots inside the front door. Her straight brown hair, parted in the center, hung below her shoulders, hippie-style. Faded and patched blue jeans and a loose red plaid man's shirt completed her perception of a cool college student's attire. She believed in God, but not in Jesus.

Just a few years earlier, her younger brother, Geoffrey, had been killed instantly in a car crash. Beth had turned to Kelly, a burgundy Irish setter, to help her recover from the tragedy. Now she advocated a dog for Rob, preferably an Irish setter, to help heal his wounds.

Rob maintained that if someone hadn't claimed the beautiful reddish gold animal standing between them, it would have been sent to a medical research laboratory. "I just had to take him!" he pleaded.

Our two cats demanded little attention, which suited our lifestyle, and we felt no need for a dog. But we agreed to let the setter stay, based on Rob's promise to look after it.

Realization

Hope: Believing in spite of the evidence—and watching the evidence change.[4]

The following Wednesday, Jack's sister Carol drove the 200 miles from Lookout Point to be with us. At noon, we went to the hospital cafeteria for lunch. There we met Dr. Hofmann.

Both Dr. Morello and Father Cyril were encouraging us to have someone tell John about the seriousness of his illness. After we had exchanged greetings and introductions, I said to Dr. Hofmann, "I'm not certain that we should tell John."

"No?" he said. Having withdrawn from the case, he had been noncommittal when we discussed the issue that night on the fourth floor.

I continued, "Well, Dr. Hofmann, consider yourself. When you have a dark day, hope is the only thing that gets you through it—the hope that tomorrow will be better. Considering that, then, would you want someone to tell you that you're going to have a lifetime of dark days? Would you be able to bear it?"

Looking down at the floor, he admitted, "No, I guess I'd choose the hope." Then he added, "We're putting your son in a room with a man in a circular bed who has a virus of the spinal cord. He'll be there for a year." After a pause, he continued, "But he stands a better chance of recovering than your son does."

4 Astara's Newsletter, *The Voice*, Upland, California, August 1994.

I stared at him blankly. Dr. Hofmann was trying to prepare me. According to the best medical opinions, John suffered from malignant cancer—cause unknown, and incurable.

***

That Friday morning, I awoke feeling doomed, as if I were going to the gas chamber. For that day we would learn the results of the biopsy. We would find out how long John would live, or how long before we would pray that he would die.

"Oh God, I can't go!" I cried. But a voice within overruled me. *"Oh yes, you can. Get up and get going."* Finally, I came to my senses and realized that there was nothing to lose. The biopsy would only confirm what we already knew. Bracing myself, I dressed to go to the hospital and took more extra-strength aspirin to prepare myself for the blow.

However, at the hospital, I felt dizzy and weak at the knees, unable to move from my chair—but not for the reasons anticipated. Dr. Morello pulled up a chair and sat facing us. He said that the prognosis was different from what the doctors had expected. The biopsy showed that the tumor in John's spinal cord was malignant, but it was not the kind that would spread through the body. It should respond to cobalt treatments.

Confused, I tried to sort out the message. Were they saying that John would live, after all?

"Of course, he won't be normal," Dr. Morello went on. "But if he were my boy, I would just be thankful that things turned out so much better than they might have. There's no reason why he can't continue his education."

We were speechless. Finally, I ventured, "Then let's not tell him."

Dr. Morello crossed his legs and rested his elbow on the arm of the chair. Cupping his chin in his hand, he asked, "Tell him what?"

Silence. Leaning over to make eye contact with me, he repeated coldheartedly, "Tell him what?"

Faltering, I said, "Well, you know." I could not utter that terrible word, *cancer*. I recoiled when anyone used it in regard to John. It was easier for me to accept the word *tumor*. It seemed less horrifying.

He stared at me cruelly, waiting, almost willing me to say it. I mumbled, "You know."

After another silence, I suggested, "Let's just tell him it's a tumor."

"What awful word?" he insisted.

I panicked and choked up.

"Malignant," Jack interjected.

Sneering, Dr. Morello turned away from me and sat sideways in his chair. In the early 1970s, doctors and nurses addressed the physical needs of the cancer patient, but care was sorely lacking for the psychological and emotional needs of the patient and family.

Slowly, steadily, I emphasized, "A tumor is enough to say." I feared that using the word *cancer* in front of John might intimidate him to the point that his immune system would be weakened.

The doctor stood up quickly and started toward the door. "All right," he conceded, "he's your child." As he looked back over his shoulder, however, I saw that his eyes were steel-like. "I'll look into the radiation," he said. "I don't know—we may be able to treat him here."

"Oh, I hope so," I said. "I hope we don't have to leave. They've been so kind here." I felt that the prayers at St. Luke's had helped us persevere. I didn't know then that Dr. Morello would lash out at me for this innocent statement. Only later would I learn from the nurses of the fierce competition between the administrators, the doctors, and the staff at St. Luke's and Benjamin Taylor.

***

The next day, when Dr. Hofmann was making rounds, he told John that he would have to go to Benjamin Taylor for radiation treatments "so the tumor won't come back." Earlier that day, Dr. Morello had informed

Jack that we would have to go to Benjamin Taylor for treatment because it was the only hospital in the area that had a cobalt machine.

"Of course," he added, "your wife may have a problem with it. She doesn't want to go." Just the day before, he had said that it might be possible for John to have radiation treatment at St. Luke's. I was willing to go along with that. As I saw it at this point, it would be best for John if changes in his care could be held to the absolute minimum.

"Forget it, doctor," Jack answered. "Whatever you say, we'll do." Thus, they made plans to take John by ambulance to Benjamin Taylor the following Tuesday.

On the third day after his surgery at St. Luke's, John was moved from intensive care to Med I, where he shared a room with the man in the circular bed. When I visited in the afternoon, I learned that this man's wife was the same woman who had told me not to give up hope as she sat beside me that night in the fourth-floor waiting room.

Recognizing me as I walked in, she smiled and asked, "How are things going?"

I said simply, "Better. How are things with you?"

"He's had a setback," she replied, "but he'll be all right. More mucus has collected in his throat."

That night, while waiting in the hallway for the respiratory therapist to finish treating John, I saw Dr. Hofmann in the distance taking long strides toward me. Fearing his reaction to the results of the biopsy (which reversed the prognosis he had offered), I wanted to turn and escape, but I couldn't do so gracefully; our eyes had met. I had seen proud men bristle when women knew they had erred. Bella Abzug and Gloria Steinem were much in the news in those days, and many men, especially those fifty and older, were not ready or willing to accept the creed of the feminist movement.

Before I could move, Dr. Hofmann stood in front of me. Looking down at me, he asked in a husky, emotion-packed voice, "What does the boy say?"

"He wants to be home by Thanksgiving," I replied, choosing my words carefully. I didn't want to alienate him. We needed a neurosurgeon, and I had already estranged myself from Dr. Morello.

"He ate steak tonight. We brought it to him," I told him. The staff knew that John would not eat the hospital food, and steaks were the only fare that appealed to him. I rarely cooked them at home, but high-protein diets were a fad at the time, and steak and salad were believed to be beneficial for weight loss and good health.

Dr. Hofmann did not reply. Instead, he went into the room to see the man in the circular bed. Following him, I joined Jack and John. As the doctor was leaving, he stopped by John's bed.

"Pull up your leg." He smiled at John.

John flexed the muscles in his left leg slightly.

"Now pull up your right leg," Dr. Hofmann said.

John could only wiggle the toes a little.

"All right." Dr. Hofmann nodded, and started to leave.

"Dr. Hofmann?" John called after him.

"Yes," the doctor answered softly.

"Will you move my hips a little—over this way?"

Walking back to him, Dr. Hofmann put his long fingers under the boy and lifted him over in the bed. All was quiet, and as I watched the doctor reposition my son, I felt a presence in the room.

Smiling, Dr. Hofmann asked John tenderly, "Is that all right?"

"Mmm-hmm," John replied contentedly, remarking after the doctor had left that he certainly did feel better.

***

John was in good spirits that week. He mentioned only once that he would never be able to play sports again. He addressed this comment, not to Jack and me, but to his brother. God sometimes lends a restraining hand. My husband and I had already dealt with so many issues.

"I'll never be able to play in sports again, Rob," he acknowledged wistfully.

Turning his face away from him, Rob had responded by wheeling around and kicking the leg of the bed. Finally, he said, "Now look, kid. Never mind about that. Just get well, John."

***

Weeks later, after John was able to walk through the parallel bars in physical therapy at Benjamin Taylor, Dr. Morello issued an order that he be put back to bed. X-rays showed that his spine was curving. "One can list just from pain," the doctor explained. He suggested that we call in Dr. Cervoni, an orthopedic surgeon, to examine John.

I did not want my son to worry about the setback. One day, when we were alone, I said, "John, Dr. Cervoni told me that once you get the strength back in your legs, you won't lose it."

Relieved, John let me know for the first time that he was fully aware of his prognosis. "I heard Dr. Hofmann talking about it the day they did the myelogram," he told me.

I stared at him, speechless. Now I understood Dr. Hofmann's words that night on the fourth floor following the surgery. When we had worried about who would break the news to John about his paralysis, Dr. Hofmann had said, "Maybe we won't have to tell him." We had wondered at the time why they hadn't sedated John when they did the myelogram. Afterwards, whenever John spoke of it, it was obvious that he regarded it with horror. Although he expressed fear that he might have to repeat it, he never mentioned that he had overheard the doctors talking about him.

"The day that I had surgery," John continued, "Dr. Hofmann walked into the operating room and yelled at the anesthesiologist and the nurses, 'Do you mean to say that you're not ready when paralysis might strike at that boy lying over there any minute?' Dr. Hofmann didn't know that I was still conscious. I was supposed to be asleep by the time he arrived. Then I saw the operating table, but instead of it being flat, it was curved up in the air. I cried out, 'You aren't going to put me on that, are you?' and Dr. Hofmann came over and said that they would let it down for me."

John and I sighed simultaneously, relieved that we had finally dealt with this issue.

The Catheter

For the first three days after surgery, John eliminated by means of a catheter, a flexible, tubular instrument passed through the urethra to draw urine from the bladder. On the fourth day, he mentioned to me that the nurses had removed the catheter during the night.

"What a strange time to do it," I said. Why in the night?

Later, Dr. Morello said to Jack, "You don't know how lucky you are. If that boy hadn't been able to hold his urine, he would have walked around with a catheter in him for the rest of his life."

Apparently we were riding the edge of a dark abyss that might swallow us at any moment. Day by day, we learned that paralysis is an elusive thing, and only time would lead us to or from it.

***

Although Mr. Roberts's rare type of spinal cord virus had mysteriously disappeared, his doctors said it would be a year before he would walk. He rejected this news. A year of helplessness? Never! A man in his forties, he had never been sick a day in his life.

Nevertheless, he lay helpless in a circular bed in the room he shared with John. The bed was equipped with a mechanical device that turned it upside down to enable the strapped-in, paralyzed patient to expel mucus from his lungs. Because he was unable to push his bedside button for help, the nurses left his light on all night.

Mrs. Roberts drove fifty miles to the hospital each afternoon and stayed through the night with her husband, dozing fitfully in a chair by his bed. One day when she came in, her husband begged her to get him out of the hospital, insisting that he would go berserk if he had to stay in that bed one day longer.

She left early that evening and did not return, but I did not know why until the next afternoon, when she whispered the details to me. Although she had been devastated by her husband's outburst, she had gone away to collect herself. She said that he would get better because he had to. He had three young daughters who needed him.

That night, I sat alone with John, praying for Mrs. Roberts's husband, when a tall, broad-shouldered young man with a ruddy complexion entered the room and walked over to his bed. The man, dressed in a light gray business suit, introduced himself to Mr. and Mrs. Roberts as a faith healer.

Absorbed in my own thoughts, I paid no attention as he read Mr. Roberts passages from the Bible, but my pulse quickened when I heard him say loudly, "We don't promise any miracles, but miracles do happen!" In these secular times, scarcely anyone dared say aloud that an all-powerful Supreme Being knew of our needs and would help us if only we would ask Him.

After the faith healer had left, Mrs. Roberts came over and bent down close to me. Nodding toward her husband, she whispered, "I'm surprised! He really fell for it!" He had renewed his faith and grasped the hope that the faith healer had brought with him. Nevertheless, she said she was angry.

Surprised, I asked, "Why?"

"Because I would have preferred to call our minister," she explained. Relatives had invited the faith healer to come without her knowledge or permission. Although I said nothing, I wondered why she would care. The faith healer had strengthened her husband and given him hope. What did it matter who had accomplished it? And I thought of these words: *"Be not forgetful to entertain strangers: for thereby some have entertained angels unawares."*[5]

---

[5] Heb. 13:2

LEAVING ST. LUKE'S

Drug addiction among students was now an issue of national concern, and it was very much on my mind during my conversation with a young nurse the night before we left St. Luke's. Earlier that year, while John was a patient at Cobourg Hospital, his eyes had crossed and glazed over from taking sleeping pills. Now, following his surgery, he had received 22 hypodermic injections for pain. He told me that he looked forward to the shots, saying that they "make me feel cool." I was fearful that he had become addicted to the drugs, but the nurse reassured me. We agreed that, instead of worrying about the outcome, I should just be thankful that the medical profession had the means to relieve his pain.

At 9 p.m. I headed down the corridor to go home, but I stopped abruptly when the nurse called out after me, "I'll remember your son in my prayers."

Looking back at her, I begged, "Oh, please do. Prayers are the most important thing of all." Walking toward the front entrance to meet Jack, I realized that this team spirit at St. Luke's had given me additional strength to endure.

In the lobby, we exchanged goodbyes with Dr. Hofmann. I had left word at the desk that I wanted to see him. I needed to be reassured about going to the Benjamin Taylor. He sighed as he approached us. Here was a man spurred on by the intriguing challenge of sometimes winning, sometimes losing. He seemed to belong there as much as the pale green walls, the lonely corridors, and the wooden crucifixes.

The world inside the hospital seemed peaceful, almost like being in a monastery, with its prayers and supportive staff. By contrast, in the world outside, hate prevailed, and people were yelling at one another. Angry peace activists were in Washington to protest the Vietnam War, and civil rights advocates were promoting their cause just as vociferously.

"We hate to be transferred, Dr. Hofmann," I said. "It's so beautiful here. Do you think we should go?"

His eyes lit up and he answered quietly, "Thank you. We like to think our patients get good care." Then, looking at me with raised eyebrows, he inquired, "You don't want to leave?"

"I can't," I said, "without the prayers. I guess we'll just have to take the prayers with us." That afternoon I had left a note in Father Cyril's mailbox, asking him to bring communion to John at Benjamin Taylor. By car, that hospital was just ten minutes away from St. Luke's.

"Dr. Hofmann, you have some beautiful people upstairs—Father Cyril and Sister Anastasia, for instance," I continued. "When you're down, they pick you right up and put you on your feet again." I wondered then how others managed to survive similar crises without prayers.

Nodding, he said, "You should go to Benjamin Taylor. We have no cobalt machine here." Then, hesitating, he warned, "The boy won't get it all back...."

Realizing that he meant that John would never walk normally again, I interrupted him. "Oh, Dr. Hofmann—please—no more bad news." I felt like a tree stump being continuously whacked with an ax.

"No?" he replied. Could I not accept it?

In the silence now between us, I thought about how much lighter his burden would be if only he had more hope—something beyond scientific data. "You should believe, Dr. Hofmann. Then you'd be more optimistic," I said.

He gazed at the floor, as if in a trance, as his mind's eye flashed hundreds of images projecting confrontations with truth that bring a man to his final conclusions. At last, he lifted his eyes, and looking into the distance, he said softly, "I do believe."

My heart leaped as I heard this proclamation of faith. His words reinforced my own faith at a time when liberal clergy were preaching from the pulpit, "Forget prayer. It's old-fashioned. Dialogue is what matters."

Dr. Hofmann took my hand and held it. In this gesture he said what words could never say. He was sorry—sorry for all the heartache we'd suffered, sorry that he did not have a remedy for it, and sorry that we'd had to endure additional pain concerning the anticipated results of the biopsy, which later turned out to be false. But I did not blame him. No one knew, as I knew, that God might have had a hand in the matter.

***

Two days before Thanksgiving, John arrived by ambulance at Benjamin Taylor with his few belongings: a Swiss calendar watch, a brown leather wallet containing a few dollar bills, and a miraculous medal that I had given him. I had purposely packed his brown leather boots, hoping to send him an indirect message that he would walk out of the hospital.

Since most of his casual clothes were well worn, I had bought him the previous day a pair of plain tan pants and a cotton plaid sport shirt to wear for the ride across town. But when I showed them to him at the hospital, he shook his head.

"Get something cool, Mom.... Don't get anything with a brand name that looks new," he mumbled.

"What do you mean, John?" I asked. How could I buy new clothes that looked old?

"Well, get jeans and a T-shirt," he said. Happy that new clothes piqued his interest, I returned the first outfit and drove around in unfamiliar Dickinson until I found a sporting goods store that carried teen-agers' clothing. This time, knowing his love of sports, I bought a football jersey and a pair of Lee blue jeans. But John took one quick look at them and then shoved them back into the bag.

"Well, what *do* you want?" I asked him, exasperated. "This will be the second time I'll have changed these!"

Looking down at his hands, he muttered something about an Army & Navy Store. I went out to find one, only to discover that even some things that looked old from the Army & Navy Store did not pass the test. John rejected the T-shirt I bought because it was in his usual size; in order to be socially correct, it had to be oversize. Finally, after one more trip to the store, he approved of my choices.

John arrived at the hospital dressed in a lavender and white tie-dyed T-shirt, with faded purple denim jeans that had been laundered repeatedly to make them look old rather than new. After much ado, John finally looked "cool."

***

Through the large window of John's room on the third floor, we could see the stars and stripes whipping on a flagpole near the hospital's emergency entrance. An electronically controlled bed replaced his bed at St. Luke's, which had been operated by hand cranks. Instead of a crucifix at the foot of the bed, there was an oil painting of a boy watching sailing vessels from the edge of a wharf in New England.

A nurse pointed out that in the new wing on the same floor, a patient could select a room with turquoise or gold wall-to-wall carpeting. The dull green walls at St. Luke's were now out of favor. Hospital interior decorators were using colors and furnishings that they believed would be psychologically beneficial to the patient.

After John had settled down in his new surroundings, Jack and I tried to rest. Discussing John's case with anyone sapped my strength, so I entered and left the hospital as inconspicuously as possible. I tried to block out of my mind all that had happened. The next six days passed uneventfully, providing us with a respite to gather ourselves. Still, I was not prepared for what happened on the following Monday morning.

As I walked down the corridor toward John's room on that snowy day, I heard a voice call out from behind me, "Mrs. Redmond?" Turning around, I saw a young, thin-faced redhead wearing a head nurse's nametag looking at me from the nurses' station.

"Yes," I said.

"Dr. Morello left a message for you this morning."

"He did? What was that?"

"He said to tell you that you can go back to St. Luke's."

I froze in my tracks. I felt as if someone had slapped me across the face. I remembered that I had praised the staff at St. Luke's in front of Dr. Morello, and I momentarily wondered if that had prompted his suggestion. He was well aware that we had to stay at Benjamin Taylor. The only other hospital in the region that offered radiation therapy was 200 miles away in Rockleigh.

Blindly, I wheeled around and groped my way along the wall into John's room, standing with my back to him to hide my frustration. Then, composing myself, I turned to my son and said, "Hi, honey. How are you today?"

Slowly turning his head toward me and grinning, he replied, "OK." Apparently, he had not overheard the conversation. Stumbling toward the chair by the window, I threw myself into it and stared blankly out at the snow.

***

A few days later, while looking through his mail, John found a get-well card with no signature. On the front of the card, a voluptuous cross-eyed lady sat at a desk in front of a typewriter. Her pencil-black hair corkscrewed out from her head, her complexion was pale green, and she wore a tight orange dress that bulged at the seams. The card read,

The doctor says your operation
didn't turn out the way he had figured.

On the inside, a middle-aged doctor wearing a bow tie, striped black and white pants, and brown and white shoes held a stethoscope in his hand. The message continued:

It didn't quite pay for his new yacht!
(Get Well Soon!)

A handwritten note scrawled at the bottom of the card said,

This place isn't quite what it used to be.
Hurry back!

The lack of a signature puzzled me, but John knew right away that the card had come from the nurses at St. Luke's. Since it had been addressed to Benjamin Taylor, a rival hospital, they had not dared to sign it. But they wanted John to know that they, too, reveled in his glorious victory. The results of the biopsy, which contradicted the expectations of the doctors, indicated that John would walk with a cane instead of being confined to a wheelchair.

REVELATION

As she watched me, when I was a young girl playing on the kitchen floor with Buddy, my black and white terrier, my Aunt Kate would often exclaim, "My, Barbara, you look like your father!"

John's namesake—my father—John Marston, died in 1965. He had married my mother when he was nineteen and she was eighteen. After migrating to the United States from Wolfe Island, one of the Thousand Islands in Canada, both of them became naturalized citizens.

Dad was six feet tall, lean, and dark-haired. His adventurous brown eyes danced from behind dark horn-rimmed glasses. He rarely showed anger, yet those same eyes could be stern when he was disciplining me. Although he was strong as an ox, he could be as gentle as a summer breeze rippling a field of daisies. With the help of my brothers, he raised wheat, hay, and corn on part of our 150-acre dairy farm, using the non-tillable soil as pasture for the Holsteins and workhorses.

Starting his day at 5 a.m., he and one of my brothers milked the cows, then dumped the pails of warm milk into covered steel cans in a large, iced vat in the milk house. On occasion, my mother performed this chore in my brother's absence. By 6:30, men in the Dairymen's League Cooperative trucks picked up the ten-gallon milk cans and took them to the factory where the milk was pasteurized before it was delivered to consumers.

Because farming, then as now, was always subject to the vagaries of the weather, Dad could not rely on it alone for his livelihood. Therefore, by 7 a.m., he was at one of our two local paper mills, where he worked as a master mechanic, supervising the maintenance of heavy equipment.

Back home at 4:30 p.m., he started the evening milking. Since the cows had to be milked twice a day every day of the year, vacations were out of the question. But he must have had job satisfaction because, in later life, he told me adamantly, "If only I can keep my health, I want to work till I die."

In spite of his busy schedule, Dad's life was simple. In those days, honor was revered, and Dad trusted everyone. He sealed a business transaction with his word and a handshake. There was no need for paperwork. Fair and just as a mediator, he insisted on hearing both sides of a story before he made a decision. He would offer help to anyone who asked for it. He even found time to be a trustee of the one-room elementary school that my sister and I attended. My sister-in-law taught all eight grades there.

Dad kept abreast of current events by reading the evening newspaper and listening to a Lowell Thomas newscast on the radio. On Friday nights, he and my mother often square-danced with friends, who included our family doctor and his wife, and a couple who owned a grocery store in nearby Greenville.

On Sundays Dad listened to *The Amos and Andy Show* early in the evening, then played cards, usually pedro or euchre, with my mother and invited relatives. To my recollection, every night before he went to bed, he knelt down beside his chair in the living room and prayed the rosary.

When I was nineteen, Dad developed asthma after a long bout with bronchitis, and he could no longer tolerate the harsh northern winters. Thus, he, my mother, and I lived in the South for four years, returning home only in the summer.

Once again enjoying good health in the warmer climate, Dad worked for a plumbing contractor, supervising work in the hotels that were being constructed along Miami Beach. Long before anyone had heard of the civil rights movement, he dialogued with blacks on the job, and he often told me how he admired their easygoing manner, wry wit, and love of laughter.

Years later, with my sons John and Christopher in the back of our station wagon, I drove 150 miles almost every weekend for more than a year to be with Dad during his last illness.

Although he never put it into words—it was not the practice in those days—I always knew that he loved me. He discussed world affairs with me, and by listening and talking with me in an adult manner, he gave me stability. He was my rock, and when that great piece of granite crumbled, I fought his death. It was my first encounter with that dreadful menace that takes our loved ones away from us.

What I lamented was the permanence of death. I would never see my father again. Never! Oh, yes, theologians said that there was a hereafter, but they had not been there and seen it. No one was certain.

Finally, after a year of tormenting myself over Dad's death, our good family doctor, Dr. O'Bryan, uttered just two words that snapped me out of it. "Barbara," he said, "accept it!" I had not realized how much I had been fighting Dad's departure until that moment. Nor did I know that, later in life, I would have a painful experience that would change my perception of death forever.

***

One year later, I discovered a pea-sized lump on the side of my breast. Warily, I made an appointment with Dr. Martino, a surgeon. "Probably benign," he said, "but you never know. Have it removed." Having been hospitalized only for childbirth, I'd had no experience with surgery. Hugging Jack and the children, I told them, "Don't worry. I'll be home in three or four days. Insignificant!"

That September afternoon, I entered Cobourg Hospital, frightened but determined that this surgery would have a positive outcome. It had to. I had four young children. Back in my room the next day, when nurses roused me after the surgery, I thanked God that it was over and snuggled down into my pillow.

The next morning, Dr. Martino, a tall, broad-shouldered man in his early fifties, looked in on me. "You don't have anything rushing on, Mrs. Redmond, do you? At home, I mean."

"Why, no, not really," I replied as I thought of my three boys between the ages of thirteen and four, wrestling, giggling, and chasing each other after school from the kitchen to the dining room to the living room to the hall and back to the kitchen again. I shrugged. Jack would just have to leave work early and stay with them so they wouldn't kill one another.

"Well, why don't you just stick around for a few days and rest?" the doctor advised. "I'm going fishing, and when I come back, I'll see you."

"Well, it's all right with me," I said. How kind of Dr. Martino to let me have a little rest before I went home. Like any full-time mother who worked fourteen hours a day, seven days a week, I welcomed the prospect of sleeping in and having my meals served to me.

On the third day, Dr. Martino's associate, Dr. Foster, greeted me. "Mrs. Redmond, how are you this morning?"

"Fine, just fine," I beamed.

"I understand you're staying until we find out for sure if your tumor is malignant," he said matter-of-factly.

Rising in the bed, I replied, "You...understand...WHAT?"

"Malignant. It might be malignant," he said. He added that I might have to have a radical mastectomy. It would take about three days to obtain the results of the biopsy.

Horrified, I sank into the bed and pulled the sheets up around my neck.

When the doctor had left, I telephoned Jack with the news. He was so overwhelmed that he turned to a friend to help him compose himself before he attempted to face me. Meanwhile, I lay curled up in my bed, alone, petrified. And for five consecutive hours, I prayed the rosary.

About 4 p.m. that day, Dr. Martino came to my room and stood just inside the door. He called out heartily across the room, "Mrs. Redmond, I'm back!"

"You are?" I lay frozen, not daring to turn my head to look at him.

"Sure. You can go home!"

I sat up in bed. "I can what?"

"You're OK! You can go home!"

"Was...it...?" I couldn't finish the question.

"No, but I would have sworn it was malignant! It sure looked like it to me! I can hardly believe that it wasn't!" Looking down, he scraped the toe of his deerskin shoe along the floor.

Neither could I. His good news overwhelmed me.

During this time, I had become aware that a patient often felt abandoned in such circumstances. It was almost as if he or she had leprosy. Few could offer help. Everything was so frightening. Loved ones, unable to contain their horror and grief, would not come by to visit. Doctors stood at the door to deliver a message, then made a quick exit. Nurses continued to provide care, but now they seemed to choose each word carefully lest they betray their emotions. As a result, the patient faced a double predicament: an uncertain medical future and no one to allay his or her fears.

When the good news finally came, I picked up the pieces of my shattered psyche and called home. "Come and get me," I begged weakly.

***

In 1968, when John was eleven, Martin Luther King was assassinated, and civil disobedience seemed to be everywhere. God, the American flag, motherhood, and apple pie were out of favor.

At that time, one of the issues in the civil rights movement was interracial marriage. Some declared that the white man's rejection of this concept was causing the mounting tension between the two races.

As a published freelance writer, I had penned what seemed to be a solution to the conflict. I pointed out in my article that results from a recent survey showed that the majority of blacks did not support interracial marriage. Instead, they preferred to preserve their own culture and heritage. "In addition," I concluded, "God must have wanted blacks to be black, or he wouldn't have made them that way." Since timeliness was important, I hurried the piece off to an editor.

However, a few days later, after envisioning hosts of angry whites and blacks shaking their fists at me, I reconsidered. Even in my quiet northern town with its small black population, tempers flared if this topic was even mentioned in a church sermon. Violence was always a possibility, and I was afraid. I did not want to be shot. Therefore, I prayed that my article would promptly hit the wastebasket when it arrived on the editor's desk.

Ordinarily, an editor returns a rejected manuscript within five or six weeks. In this instance, however, six months passed and I still had no reply. I breathed easier. This article would have required immediate publication in order to be effective.

When the large brown envelope finally appeared in the mailbox, I handled it as if it were a time bomb. The entire afternoon had gone by before I could muster up the courage to open it. Inside, I found the manuscript and an attached note from the editor. In it, he apologized, saying that he did not understand how it had happened, but he had found the article only that day, buried under some papers. I gratefully accepted his rejection notice.

During this long period of waiting, I had feared for my safety. What if my manuscript were published? I worried. While praying about it one day, I heard sounds like the echo of footsteps behind me, and from the depths within me, a female voice whispered, *"Why are you afraid? Didn't I pull you out of trouble when you were in the hospital?"* Although I told no one about this incident, I knew that our Blessed Mother had spoken to me.

I had gasped when I recalled my hospital stay three years earlier. That time, too, I had begged God to save me. Even before he had seen the results of the biopsy, Dr. Martino felt certain that my tumor was malignant. But it wasn't! Had this, then, been more than coincidence?

That was the reason why, years later, I had asked Dr. Hofmann a second time if he was sure that John's tumor was malignant. I knew that he had not yet seen the results of the biopsy. He insisted then that his view would prove to be correct, adding that Dr. Morello was in complete agreement.

After remembering the agony I had endured before the first about-face, I knew that I didn't want any more shocks like that one. On second thought, however, I decided that I shouldn't complain about a shock that conveyed such welcome news.

Father, Father, Where Are You?

Only one priest brought communion to John in the first three weeks, but I could do little about it. All choked up, I could not talk on the telephone, and I refused to take calls at home. Friends, understanding, talked to Jack, who relayed their messages to me. Prayers uplift and strengthen the spirit, but now, at Benjamin Taylor, our burden increased as the prayers dwindled.

Every day, I believed that Father Cyril would come to see us. Before we left St. Luke's, I had asked him to visit my son in his new hospital. At that time, I had also written a note to Sister Anastasia:

> *Dear Sister Anastasia,*
>
> *How can I thank you for your kindness that terrible night up on the fourth floor? That night, we went home and prayed for a miracle because a miracle was all we had left to pray for.*
>
> *After we had endured three days and nights of agony, believing there was no hope, the doctors said that John does have a malignancy in the spinal cord, but it should respond to cobalt radiation. It is not the kind that spreads through the body. We have to transfer to Benjamin Taylor tomorrow, but in this atheistic world, I am afraid to go.*
>
> *I'm asking Father Cyril to come over there to see John.*

I was uninformed about hospital procedures, but I assumed that, on request, the chaplain of one hospital would bring Holy Communion to a patient in another. Only later did I learn that this assumption was incorrect. This must have been the reason Father Cyril did not come.

At the end of the third week at Benjamin Taylor, I felt a hand touch my shoulder as I was sipping coffee in the snack bar. Whirling around on my stool, I was surprised to see Marty Donegan standing behind me. A long-time friend, she was now a guidance counselor in the hospital's school of nursing.

"What are you doing here?" she inquired.

"John's here."

"How come? What's wrong?"

"He's been transferred here from St. Luke's."

"What for?"

"Radiation."

"Where?"

"Spinal cord."

Marty's face turned ashen, but I quickly reassured her. "No, Marty. We feel good about it. It's turned out better than we expected." Remembering her claim that she had revived her young daughter with prayers when she was close to death during a serious illness, I felt safe in adding, "John's being healed by prayer."

Marty nodded.

"But I can't find a priest, Marty," I continued. "I don't know any priests in Dickinson."

"I do," she said. "I'll call one right away. Father McMahon—he's a beautiful man. He's about forty-five or fifty, conservative. He's at St. Raphael's. He used to be chaplain at St. Luke's. You'll like him."

Then, angrily, she added, "These priests these days! Where are they? I can't believe it! They should be here with the sick. We shouldn't have to call them! It's a good thing we still have our own relationship with God, or we'd have nothing!" I nodded in agreement.

Marty had to get back to work, but as we bade each other goodbye, she reassured me that she would call Father McMahon as soon as she returned to her office.

But the weekend passed, and he failed to appear. I took a deep breath, choked back the lump in my throat, and dialed the operator for his number. Perhaps he had simply forgotten.

When he answered the phone, I stuttered, "F-F-Father McMahon? You don't know me, but my friend, Marty Donegan, told me about you. She called you last week about bringing my son communion at Benjamin Taylor. He's very ill, Father."

In a low, husky voice, he said, "No, I received no call."

"No call at all? She didn't call you, Father?"

"No. I received no call," he repeated.

I hesitated. "Well, perhaps she couldn't get you. Perhaps you were out. But anyway, Father, I need a priest to come and see my son at Benjamin Taylor. Last week, he had a serious operation. Father, you probably won't believe this, but prayers are carrying him through!" I was almost afraid to say this even to a priest, for I'd heard that some priests were ridiculing the blind faith of the layperson.

"Why of course I believe you," Father McMahon said. "I had cancer myself last spring, and I honestly believe it was prayers that made me better."

I had cancer myself! I hadn't told him that my son had cancer. When referring to John, I still couldn't say it!

In disbelief, I repeated, "You had cancer last spring, Father, and you're better?"

"Yes, of course," he asserted. "I told the doctor right out that I wanted to know the truth, and he told me I had it."

There was a dramatic pause. Cancer was terminal—everyone knew that—yet this was the third person I'd heard of in the religious community who claimed to have recovered from cancer. The religious, by nature, would turn to prayer for their healing. Was this significant?

Father McMahon was still recuperating, and so he could not come to see John. But he promised to send his assistant, Father Santo. Later, I learned that Marty had left a message for Father McMahon with his housekeeper, who had forgotten to tell him.

***

Father Santo seemed to be in a rather exuberant mood when he came into John's room. Unfortunately for him, he encountered an extremely anxious mother who had been keeping a lonely three-week vigil with a sick child. During that time, my emotions had been all bottled up inside me. By now, I was a boiling volcano ready to erupt.

"Well, Father Santo," I started, "I'm so glad you've come. It's been such a long time since a priest has been in…."

The young priest nodded and turned to John. "I'm Father Santo," he said as he searched for the name card at the head of the bed. "Are you John?"

I interrupted before John could answer. "Father, it's a shame that this hospital doesn't have a chaplain. A priest should be here with the sick at all times."

Eyes blazing, I continued, "It strikes me as odd, Father, that in these times a church member can receive communion every Sunday only if he is well enough to go to church, but he can't receive communion at all if he is sick and his need for it is even greater. After all, Father, Christ is the healer of the sick, isn't he?"

When he didn't answer, I repeated, "*Isn't he, Father?*"

Tightening his nostrils and pursing his lips, Father Santo backed away. He had not expected to run into an argument on this good-will mission. Narrowing his small blue eyes behind his wire-rimmed glasses, he said, "Well, now, I don't know. I wouldn't say that…."

"Well I would!" I shot back. "Where are all our priests anyway? Out politicking?" As I saw the blood rush up from his collar, past his ears to his dark hairline where the roots of his hair were noticeably bristling, I stopped. His eyes expressed shock.

What had I said, I wondered, that had so upset him? I assumed that he was conservative, like Father McMahon, so I was not singling *him* out. I was directing my anger at priests collectively.

Weeks later, I read in the morning newspaper that Father Santo was a leader in the Diocesan Ecumenical Movement. I supported this movement on the premise that all Christians, regardless of their denomination, were praying to the same God. I also approved of other changes being considered within the Church. But the fact remained that some young liberal priests, overly consumed with social and political issues, were neglecting the sick, who desperately needed them.

Instead of praying over John, Father Santo gave a short sermon to the effect that we were gathered there to be with John in his time of illness. He neither gave John his blessing nor made the sign of the cross over his head, as was the custom. He brought communion on one other occasion. Then we never saw him again.

So once more I turned to Marty, who located Father Bonacci. A former missionary priest, he was now an assistant at St. Peter's. He came regularly to see John, bringing much-needed strength and comfort to both my son and me, until he was stricken with influenza at holiday time.

Another Time-Same Circumstances

One day, when I returned from the snack bar, John and his roommate were talking about steaks—still John's favorite food. I continued to take broiled steaks to him four or five times a week for his evening dinner, reasoning that the protein would keep his strength up. His roommate, a gray-haired man with a brush cut, peered over at me through silver-rimmed glasses. "Every time I cook a steak, I burn it!" he joked.

Throwing my coat on the chair, I whirled around and faced him. "I'll bet your wife can cook it just right!" I said teasingly.

His wan smile faded. Shaking his head, he said, "Oh no. My wife's in Elmview." Although Elmview was an expensive nursing home that had just opened in the area, I had heard that its performance ratings ranged from mediocre to low.

Curious, I asked, "Does she like it there?"

"Oh, she doesn't know she's there," he said. His countenance saddened, and I regretted that I had mentioned her to him. But then it occurred to me, *If she doesn't know she's there, then she doesn't know he's here!* Who was looking after him? I had seen only one elderly woman visit him since his arrival.

Drawing his bushy gray eyebrows down in a frown, he continued, "My doctor hasn't come in to report on my X-rays. He told me he would be in this morning, but he didn't show up."

At that moment two Cobourg priests, Father O'Donnell and Father Schosger, looked in. They called out to John across the room, "Hi, how are you today?" Father Schosger had visited us at Cobourg Hospital, but when I had asked him to bring John communion, he had refused, saying that he brought communion only to dying patients.

Conservative Father O'Donnell, a dark-haired, blue-eyed Irishman in his early fifties, believed that left-wing clergymen were misleading parishioners and bringing about the collapse of the church. I had recently read one of his articles on the new role of the parish priest in the diocesan newspaper.

That role, he had stated, was not as complex as some would like to make it. On the contrary, it was the same as it had always been: to say Mass, to teach children, to visit the sick, and to administer the Sacraments. "These duties will take up most of his time if the priest does them well," he contended.

After greeting me, the two priests walked over to John and gave him their blessing.

On the way out, Father O'Donnell, nodding to John's roommate, asked, "Has your pastor been in?"

"Oh, no." The old man shook his head, seemingly embarrassed.

"Why not?" Father O'Donnell continued.

"Oh," the man shrugged, "I don't believe he even knows I'm here."

"Why not? Doesn't he make rounds at the hospital?"

"I don't know."

"What parish do you belong to?"

"St. Casmir's."

Father O'Donnell nodded. After giving the man their blessing, the two priests departed.

Within the next half-hour, a man dressed in an olive coat, olive trousers, and red plaid sport shirt came in and introduced himself to John's roommate as Father Mansell from St. Casmir's.

"How did you know I was here?" the old man asked.

"Father O'Donnell called me. I didn't know you were here," the priest shrugged.

The next morning, John's roommate went home.

THE LAND OF TECHNOLOGY

On the day that John began radiation therapy, Jack had to meet with a corporate executive to discuss the second phase of his house plans. Since electrical contracting was his livelihood, he did not feel he could cancel the meeting. Thus, I went to the hospital alone. Science had never been my forte. I had little interest in it. It seemed so cold and methodical. So it was not surprising to me that the radiology department looked like a death chamber.

When I returned to John's room after lunch, a pleasant, dark-haired nurse told me that Dr. Rodriguez wanted to see me. I acknowledged her with a smile but did not answer. I did not want to see the doctor, although I knew that I should stay with John for moral support. Therefore, when they rolled John onto the gurney to take him to the X-ray department, I followed, feeling like a lamb being led to slaughter.

I sat in the waiting room until a young radiologist came to escort me down the hall. Taking long strides in his brown leather boots, he spoke excitedly about the hospital's computer hookup for terminal cancer patients. To the average person, computers were as foreign as objects from outer space, to be used only by technical experts.

As we passed an open door leading into the room where John lay on a black examining table, I cautioned the radiologist, "Shhh! The boy doesn't know what he has!"

"Oh," he replied.

I didn't understand why he was so excited about hooking up the computers. It didn't excite me. *This was my son, a real person with feelings, that he was talking about. Didn't he realize that?* Trying to reassure me, he explained that they would determine by computer the correct amount of cobalt to use. But that did not comfort me. *Didn't he think I knew the dangers of radiation—that radium burned good cells as well as bad ones?*

Actually, at that time, I was not well informed on that subject. I did not know that only the bad cells were destroyed. The good cells that were burned had the ability to repair themselves.

A nurse joined us. She led me down the hall past the rooms with the giant X-ray machines. To my mind, in such bleak surroundings, we could have been touring a nuclear plant. To me, it looked like death's doorway.

Finally, we reached the office of Dr. Rodriguez, head of radiation therapy.

My eyes blurred with emotion. Through the haze, I saw a man in a brown jacket, and I heard a voice say, "Good afternoon, Mrs. Redmond. I'm Dr. Rodriguez. I want to explain to you about the cobalt treatments."

I shrank back. An explanation would only make me more fearful. "That's all right, Dr. Rodriguez," I said. "You don't have to…."

"Oh, but I must. I want you to know it. I want you to know that we will do everything that we can for your son, but…."

This was it. I knew it.

"I want to tell you about the side effects of radiation."

I hushed the doctor, nodding toward the open door. "He doesn't know all about it, you know," I protested.

Stepping in front of me, with his back toward the room where John lay waiting, he said quietly, "That's what I understand. He just knows he's going to be treated for a tumor?"

I took a deep breath and nodded.

"Well, that's all right. We can go along with that," he said.

I exhaled. This man was human. Curious now, my bleary eyes cleared. Taking a better look at him, I saw a man in his fifties, of medium stature, with dark brown curly hair. His compassionate eyes were sincere. My head cleared, and I understood then that he just wanted to acquaint me with the hospital's procedures. I preferred, however, to have him spare me the agony of an explanation and just get on with it.

Glancing around his office, I saw, behind his desk, a wall of X-rays with grotesque pictures of black knobs forming spines and ribs with no flesh. It was frightening. Were they John's?

Not understanding my uneasiness in surroundings in which he felt so comfortable, the doctor ventured cheerfully, "We can put your son on the television set in my office, and you can watch him while he's under the cobalt machine."

Again I shrank away. As a young girl, I had fainted at the sight of blood when I had a nosebleed.

"And we'll have to tattoo your son." He said it loud enough so that John could hear him in the next room.

"You'll have to WHAT?" I repeated, whispering.

"Tattoo your son—tattoo his back," he said.

Dumfounded, I stared at him.

"Oh," he laughed, "they'll be little pencil marks at each corner of the area where he receives radiation because he can never be given radiation there again. You see, the bone marrow...."

"Oh," I smiled. "I'm glad you explained."

Motioning toward the room where John lay, I whispered, "He's listening." Then I continued, "It took three days to convince him that the scar on his back didn't look like jagged, distorted facial scars on the monster men he'd seen on television. Even though we described the scar to him as a slightly red, thin, straight line about eight inches long, he wouldn't listen. It finally took a nineteen-year-old blonde nurse's aide to convince him that we had given him an accurate description of it."

Dr. Rodriguez laughed, but I choked back tears. Taking on a more serious expression, he said, "You must be frightened, and so must he. I understand."

Through the open door, he beckoned to a nurse, who took me out into the hall. Thankful that the introduction was over, I sank into one of the red plastic chairs lined up against the wall and began the long wait. After an hour, a nurse reassured me, "It doesn't always take this long. It's just the first day, when they do the simulation, that takes so much time."

Finally, Dr. Rodriguez came down the hall. Standing over me, he said, "One more thing I have to explain. There may be side effects from the radiation. There may be burned tissue, although we try for as little as possible, and we have to be careful of bone marrow. We'll probably treat him for four weeks. We'll consult with the University of Rockleigh. They have a computer on campus, and we'll decide what his dosage should be."

On hearing this, I broke into sobs and buried my face in my hands. *Oh, God*, I thought, *isn't there anyone anywhere who can give us peace of mind—anyone who can tell us that he will get better? Must we walk a tightrope all the way?*

Dr. Rodriguez sat down in the chair next to me. "Oh, well, now," he said. His voice softening, he continued, "This is one case we should be able to cure."

I continued sobbing.

Rising quickly, he went back to his office. A dark-haired nurse came to me and suggested that I go down to the snack bar and have some coffee.

"I guess I'll have to," I replied. I didn't want John to see me crying.

"Don't worry," she said softly. "We'll take care of him. We'll take him back to his room."

That night after dinner, when I saw the limp, uncomplaining figure in the bed searching my face for reassurance, I said, "Don't worry, honey. Everything will be all right."

The next day, Dr. Rodriguez told me that they would treat John for five weeks instead of four. He explained that by administering the maximum dosage over a longer period of time, they would minimize the side effects of the radiation.

THE FIRST CRISIS

Coping with radiation was trying, but dealing with Dr. Morello was even more difficult. In the first week, he ordered tranquilizers for John to counteract the nausea. At first, John felt sick after lunch, but by the time hospital aides had taken him down for treatment, he was fine. He was in good spirits, and unaware of the seriousness of his illness. When orderlies pushed him down the hall on a gurney and he passed nurses and other orderlies that he recognized, he often yelled to them, "Hey, they're gonna give me a shot of CO-BALT today!"—much as if they were going to give him a chocolate ice cream cone or take him to a movie.

It was hard sometimes to understand his innocence. He was an avid science student, and he never missed the television series *Medical Center*. But at that time cancer was not openly discussed in any medium. While John was in traction in Cobourg Hospital, whenever *Medical Center* flashed on the screen, Rob would call out in a singsong manner, "Hey, John, there's your favorite program!" Since Rob and his father watched sports programs almost exclusively, Rob could not comprehend John's TV choices. Lynn favored mysteries such as Perry Mason, and I, preferring to read, had no favorite program.

Staring at the perforated white squares in the ceiling, John would answer dryly, "Yeah! I thought it would be cool to be in the hospital, but it's not. There's one thing they don't tell you on *Medical Center*."

"What's that, John?" Rob prodded.

"They don't show you the pain...." Swallowing hard and long, he tried to fight back the tears.

But John had an indomitable spirit, and when he was knocked down, he always got right up again. Therefore, when they gave him tranquilizers at Benjamin Taylor, he seemed like a stranger to us—lifeless, apathetic, yielding. If we had said, "John, we're going to take you down to the morgue today and leave you there," he probably would not have reacted. Day and night, he was nauseated, unable to retain even fluid.

Although I accompanied John for his daily treatment, one afternoon I arrived at the hospital a little late. As I entered the lobby, two aides were wheeling him off the elevator. One of the aides, a rosy-cheeked, plump young woman, looked at me compassionately. With tears in her eyes, she said, "They couldn't treat him today."

Surprised, I asked, "They couldn't? Why not?"

She rolled her eyes. "This poor kid is s–i–c–k! Dr. Rodriguez said he wouldn't treat him today. He said he'd wait until he feels better."

John had been vomiting for three or four consecutive days, but when I questioned it, the nurses assured me that it was normal for nausea to accompany radiation. I assumed, therefore, that John would just have to bear it.

When I went upstairs the next day, the nurses and aides were again concerned. Dr. Morello had made the rounds that morning, but he had not changed the medication. The head nurse, who had just helped John through another vomiting session, suggested, "Why don't you call Dr. Morello?"

I hedged, saying, "Oh, I don't want to bother him on a Saturday afternoon." In truth, I really did not want to talk to him.

"Go on," she urged. "Call him at home. I'll give you the number. He won't mind."

Reluctantly, I dialed the number. When he answered, I started, "Dr. Morello? This is Mrs. Redmond. I'm calling about John. I'm so worried...."

"Worried? What about? He's fine. I saw him this morning."

"Fine? Dr. Morello.... No, I mean, he's been vomiting for four straight days and nights now. He's too weak and thin to stand radiation. Dr. Rodriguez won't treat him. He told me he was going to call you. Did he?"

"Humph! Well, yes. He told me the nausea wasn't from the radiation. But anyway, Mrs. Redmond, how can you believe that kid? He just told me this morning that he was fine!"

I paused. *Surely the doctor had looked at his charts. Hadn't the nurses told him about the nausea? He hadn't talked to me about it, although I was there every day. This man was a neurosurgeon—a specialist. We were counting on him to handle it.* His words echoed in my mind: *"How can you believe that kid?"*

"Oh, Dr. Morello," I laughed. "That's just John. He'll never admit that he isn't feeling good. Maybe he thinks it's unmanly or something. His father is like that, too. Dr. Morello, I think John is just scared. He's been through so much. Maybe it's just a self-preservation tactic."

"Well, it's hard to deal with a kid like that."

"But that's the way he is, Dr. Morello. We'll just have to accept it and take it from there. He's so sick! Dr. Morello, could we take John off the tranquilizers? I don't think they agree with him. He's vomited more since he started taking them."

"Well, all right, if you want. I'll cancel all medication."

"Well, not all medication, Dr. Morello. John needs the pain pills that you ordered. He takes them in the night, and he says they make him feel better."

"All right. I'll just cancel the tranquilizers."

"Thank you, Dr. Morello. Goodbye."

The next day, I was shocked to learn from the head nurse that Dr. Morello had canceled all medication. I stayed at the hospital ten hours that day, although we usually changed shifts when Jack came at 7 p.m. The nurses and I took turns holding John's weak, limp body up on the side of the bed for a minute to relieve the vomiting. When Jack and I left at 10 p.m., the head nurse assured us that she would call Dr. Morello if John needed a pain pill. We drove home, apprehensive.

When the nurse called Dr. Morello in the night to reissue the order for the pain pills, he complied, but he also reissued the order for the tranquilizers.

After learning this on Sunday morning, I urged John not to take the tranquilizers, but he said that he had to take them. The nurses were required to stand and wait until he swallowed them.

I realized then that only Dr. Morello had the authority to make any changes. That Sunday, the vomiting continued, and again I stayed at the hospital for ten hours. Dr. Morello had stopped in early that morning to see John, but he had made no changes in the orders.

When we went to radiation therapy on Monday, Dr. Rodriguez came out of his office and sat down beside me. "Why don't you call Dr. Morello and get him off the tranquilizers?" he urged me. "The tranquilizers may not agree with him. I know he's not nauseated from the radiation. I've told Dr. Morello that it can't be from that. He's only had a small dosage."

"I agree with you, Dr. Rodriguez," I said. "I, too, think that it's the tranquilizers. John wasn't really nauseated until he started taking them. But I asked Dr. Morello on Saturday to discontinue them, and he won't do it." I did not repeat our entire conversation, however.

Assuming that it was a misunderstanding, Dr. Rodriguez urged me, "Call him again. This boy has had a traumatic experience. If this vomiting continues, he could develop an ulcer—all sorts of things. This is serious."

Without sounding spiteful, how could I explain that I found it difficult to talk with Dr. Morello? I took a long, hard swallow. "Dr. Rodriguez, the mark of a great man in medicine is when he displays the ability to stand up and admit he is wrong. For a doctor to insist that he is right at the cost of making the patient suffer is cruel!" My eyes flashed bitterly as I thought of the doctor, who, like a headstrong captain with an uneasy crew, refused to issue a countermanding order.

Dr. Rodriguez narrowed his eyes, understanding. "I'll see what I can do," he said. "I'll talk to him." He rose from his chair and went down the hall to where John lay on a gurney, with only a few strands of blond hair showing above the sheet that covered his shadowy frame.

Bending over him, Dr. Rodriguez stroked his head, pushed his hair back out of his eyes, and said quietly, "John, when I was just your age, I found out that for the rest of my life I would be a diabetic. I was very sick, like you, John, and very discouraged, just like you are. But do you know what that made me do, John? It made me stand up and fight. It made me want to know more about diabetes—what caused it, and what could be done to prevent it. Do you know, John, it made me want to be a doctor. And now, as a doctor, I know how the other guy feels. I know how you feel, John."

John's limp body stirred feebly, and two dark-circled eyes peered out from under the sheet. Two legs pulled up, showing slight signs of life. Two whitish lips curled up at the corners.

"I'm not going to treat you today, John," Dr. Rodriguez continued, stroking John's head. "I'm not going to treat you until you feel better." Then, turning to the young aide beside him, he directed, "Take him back to his room."

In bed later that night, John smiled and said that he thought he felt better. The days dragged by, however, and another weekend passed. Under Dr. Morello's orders, John was still on tranquilizers.

THE SECOND CRISIS

One day, Dr. Morello came in and said, "I might have to put a brace on John's back." Glancing at John, I swallowed hard. The previous day, the X-ray technicians had sneaked sympathetic glances at him as they lifted him from the bed to the stretcher. John had always been lean, but now, having lost thirty pounds, he was painfully thin, weak, and helpless. He still did not complain, however.

Dr. Morello continued, "The X-rays show a slight curvature. We should have an orthopedic surgeon look at him. Whom would you like?"

"Who is there?" I asked.

He reeled off four or five names, but I did not recognize any of them. When I asked about Dr. Ferreira, he said that it would be difficult for a Cobourg doctor to handle a case in Dickinson. Finally, I chose a name that I was familiar with—Dr. Cervoni—although I did not know him personally.

When I came into John's room the next morning, the doctor had just finished examining him. Dr. Cervoni was in his late forties and of medium stature. He also turned out to be easygoing and likable.

After we had greeted each other, he said, "I can't see putting a brace on him." Hoping that he wouldn't say that dreaded word, *cancer*, in front of John, I intimated that John did not know all the details of his illness. Seeming to catch on, the doctor continued, "He may just be listing from pain."

Oh, God, thank you, I muttered under my breath.

"What did you say?"

"Nothing."

"Well, we'll just put him in a non-weight-bearing position. He can sit but not stand. We'll have the physical therapist come up here and give him exercises in bed, instead of having him go down there."

Twice a day, nurses and orderlies had been taking John to physical therapy, where he crossed the room with a walker. However, the painful procedure of rolling him onto a stretcher to take him there pulled on the incision in his back, and he had come to dread the therapy sessions.

As Dr. Cervoni started to leave, he said, "I'll tell you, from what I hear, this is a very complicated case. I wouldn't begin to scratch the surface of it."

Then, with an amused look, he continued, "By the way, I hear you want to go back to St. Luke's."

I must have looked startled, but I said nothing. *Who had told him—Dr. Morello?* Why, I wondered, did the mere mention of St. Luke's have such an abrasive effect on Dr. Morello? I had assumed that doctors liked to work together to accomplish their goals.

Just a few weeks earlier, I had vowed not to mention that hospital again. Apparently not aware that thirteen-year-old boys liked to tease, Dr. Morello had confronted John about telling the nurses that he got better care at St. Luke's. With his six-foot-three frame towering over the bedridden boy, Dr. Morello had inquired, "What's wrong that you don't like it here, John?"

Frightened, John had shrunk down in the sheets. "Why, n-n-nothing," he stuttered.

"Well, if there's anything you don't like here, let me know. I hear that you're complaining." With that, the doctor had turned and left the room.

When I had heard John say that day that he got better care at St. Luke's, I was embarrassed by it, but I joined in the laughter with the nurses as they kidded him right back. We had laughed about it again later out in the hall. The nurses weren't offended by it. They were happy to see John upbeat and talkative.

But the story had taken on a life of its own, and by the time it reached Dr. Morello, it was as if John had slandered the hospital. When we were alone later, I asked him, "How come you told them that, John?"

"Because, they'll do a lot more for me if they think they're not as good as St. Luke's," he reasoned.

"But it doesn't work that way, John," I said. "Praise works miracles. It's much better than criticism to get what you want."

Now, Dr. Cervoni's words came back to me: *I hear you want to go back to St. Luke's.* Since he practiced at both hospitals, perhaps he would not take it personally if I told him my reasons. I'd had enough of Dr. Morello's stinging innuendos.

"Yes, we liked it there," I told him quietly. "They pray there. There was love there, and they praise God. Here they praise paintings and wall-to-wall carpeting." Only then—when I had verbalized it—did I realize specifically what was lacking here. In these turbulent times, when we needed Him most, there were no outward signs of the Great Healer.

Noncommittally, Dr. Cervoni smiled and said, "Well, goodbye, Mrs. Redmond. I'll be in tomorrow." Waving to John, he went out the door.

"Goodbye, doctor," I said, deep in thought. "Yes, we'll see you tomorrow."

The Third Time

When I walked into John's room the next afternoon, he announced, "They're going to X-ray my stomach tomorrow." He was still vomiting.

I gasped, "X-ray your stomach! What for?" After the brace incident the day before, I was looking forward to a day of respite.

"I dunno."

"Who told you that?"

"Dr. Morello, when he came in this morning."

"How come?"

"Something about the pains in my sides," he shrugged.

Another sleepless night. I persuaded Jack the next morning to go with me to the hospital, but our stay was uneventful. They would not know the results of the X-rays until later in the day. We drove back home. I returned later that afternoon to accompany John to his cobalt treatment. It made me feel better to be there. I did not ask about the X-rays. I feared bad news. No one said anything to me about them.

About 4 p.m., I left the hospital and went home to get dinner for Jack and the other three children. When I arrived, I learned that Jack had gone directly from work to the hospital. When he came into the house about 9:30, he settled into his recliner to read the evening paper. Because he was so quiet, I braced myself for the blow. Facing away from him, I held onto the dining room table and asked, "How is he?"

"Oh, he's in pretty good spirits tonight," Jack said lightly.

"Does he know? Have they told him?"

"Told him what?"

"About the X-rays. Did they find anything?" I feared that they were looking for cancer in other parts of John's body.

"Why, they're all right," Jack shrugged. "Didn't you know?"

"No. No one told me. How did you find out?"

"Well, about five o'clock I went out to the desk and asked if anybody knew."

"What did they say?"

"Why, nothing. The head nurse looked at his chart and said that at ten o'clock this morning it was recorded on his chart that the X-rays were all right."

"Oh," I said wistfully. "I wish someone had told me. I've worried all day. I was afraid they'd find something else."

"Well," Jack responded, "I assumed that they'd told you."

I could not waste my diminishing energy on anger. Weakly, I put it out of my mind, went to bed, and slept well.

The next afternoon, I bounced into the hospital, cheerful—until I hit John's room.

Dully, he greeted me with, "They're going to X-ray my gall bladder tomorrow."

"Your gall bladder! What for?"

John vomited, then said, "I dunno."

"Why, John, are you sure? I can't believe it!"

"Mmm-hmm," he said, nodding. "I'm sure. Dr. Morello told me this morning."

"Told you what? What did he tell you?"

"That the X-rays yesterday showed that my stomach is touching my gall bladder."

"Oh, John. No!" They told your dad yesterday that the X-rays were fine."

For the first time, I saw a look of defeat from John. Closing his eyes, he gulped and swallowed, with tears brimming close to the surface.

"Oh, John, you're getting so weak," I protested. "You vomited all day yesterday from the barium you drank for the stomach X-rays. You're still on tranquilizers! You've had enough!"

"That's what I think," he agreed.

My tension increased as I drove home. Later that night, when I was alone, I dialed the hospital. "Give me Room 314, please."

The telephone rang repeatedly before John picked it up. He moved very slowly now.

"Hello," he said feebly.

"John?" I started.

"Yes," he replied weakly.

"Do you want to get out of that hospital or not?"

"Why, yes!" he said.

"Well, if you do, John, you had better start praying! John, you don't need anything else right now! You have enough to contend with!" In his confusion, John sometimes seemed to hope that the doctors would find something else wrong with him, reasoning that if they did, he might feel better.

"I know it," he answered.

"Well, then, you'd better start praying. You pray to God tonight that those X-rays turn out all right tomorrow." I was yelling into the phone. "You hear?"

"Y-ee-ss!" he answered.

"And John, you've lain in a fetal position for three weeks—ever since your operation." He was fearful of tearing his back incision. "It's about time you turned over on your stomach and stretched out. It's no wonder your stomach is touching your gall bladder, lying curled up in a ball like that. You hear me, John?"

"Y-ee-ss!"

"All right. Now do what I say! You hear?"

"Y-ee-ss!"

Pause.

"And John? God loves you, honey. You know we're all rooting for you."

The next morning, when I arrived at the hospital about nine o'clock, John had already been X-rayed and was back in bed, vomiting.

A compassionate young nurse attending him said, "The gall bladder X-rays didn't turn out."

Stunned, I repeated, "They didn't turn out! Why not?"

"Too much barium in his system from the stomach X-rays yesterday."

Puzzled, I asked, "Too much barium?"

"This often happens," she explained.

This often happens. "Well, that's just fine!" I exploded. "Beautiful! Don't they ever learn from their own mistakes? Certainly if it often happens, they should realize that, by waiting a day or two, the barium would have a chance to flush out of his system!"

"I know it," she shrugged.

To cool my anger, I fled from the room, went down the hall, flopped into an orange plastic-covered chair, lit a cigarette, and exhaled the blue smoke.

Looking down the hall, I saw a plump young nurse with light horn-rimmed glasses walking toward me. As she came closer, I saw the words, "HEAD NURSE" on a plastic pin on her shoulder."

"Mrs. Redmond?" she inquired.

"Yes." I shrank deeper into my chair.

"I understand that you're upset."

"Well, I am upset," I answered.

"I just came down to see if I can be of any help."

"Oh, never mind," I countered, puffing on my cigarette. "I'm angry. But I don't want to make a *big thing* about it."

"Mrs. Redmond," she went on, "I know what it's all about, and I wish I could tell you something to make you feel better, but I can't. I have to admit you're right. You have a right to be angry."

I glanced up and searched her face. She meant it.

"Well, it just seems to me," I said, trying to rationalize my anger, "that technology has become so cold and controlled that X-ray technicians don't consider they're working with *people*. They don't *see* the patients vomit for days and nights, losing sleep and getting weaker. They just sit down there with their knobs and controls and concentrate on the picture. They order the patient up and down, as if the patients were mechanical robots!"

The head nurse nodded. "That feeling has prevailed throughout this hospital for a long time, Mrs. Redmond. The medical staff has often complained about the X-ray department's lack of consideration for the patient. Many here feel that it could stand improvement."

Staring straight ahead, I nodded, deep in thought, puffing on my cigarette to soothe my frustration.

When the head nurse left and went around the corner, I overheard her saying to someone in a loud voice, "That X-ray department has been told that before. Several of the doctors have complained about it!"

At that moment, Dr. Morello stepped off the elevator and walked over to me. "How are you?" he started.

"Angry," I answered.

"What about?" He pulled up a chair beside me.

"Well, everyone reaches a breaking point, you know, and I've just reached mine."

"Why? What's the matter?"

"What's the deal on the gall bladder, Dr. Morello?" I asked.

"Well, if the stomach is touching the gall bladder, we'll have to call in another doctor," he answered.

"What kind of a doctor—a gall bladder specialist?" I said. Though I'd never heard of such a specialist, times were changing now, and it seemed as if there was a specialist for every organ in the body. I counted the doctors we had dealt with—two orthopedic surgeons, two neurosurgeons, one general practitioner for the blood clot the night of the surgery, and the head of radiation therapy. Six doctors—quite a list for someone who didn't like to change doctors.

"No, there isn't any such thing as a gall bladder specialist. Just a regular doctor."

"Oh, dear...."

"Now don't start borrowing tomorrow's troubles today," he cautioned.

Mulling it over, I said, "Well, that's right...." But still upset about the X-ray incident, I started in again. "It would have been nice, Dr. Morello, if someone had notified me yesterday about the results of John's stomach X-rays. I worried for twelve hours before I knew the outcome. The staff knew at ten o'clock yesterday morning that the results were OK, but I didn't find out until Jack told me at nine o'clock last night. What am I? Only the mother?"

"Well," Dr. Morello replied, "I can't call you at home. You have that stupid answering machine."

One time at St. Luke's, Dr. Morello had called us at home to request permission to move John to Benjamin Taylor by ambulance. When our answering machine came on, however, he left no message. Answering machines were new on the market, and callers who disliked them often left no messages. But Dr. Morello carried a pager with him at all times; he was familiar with electronic devices.

"Dr. Morello," I persisted. "You could have left word for me to call you, or directed the nurses to tell me the results of the X-rays."

Dr. Morello stood up abruptly and walked slowly to the elevator. Arriving just as it opened, he stepped on it and disappeared.

***

The next morning, while Jack and I were waiting outside the X-ray room for John, I overheard a doctor in the next room talking to the radiation technologist who had frightened me the first day. "I'm sending a patient down to you. Now don't get the man all uptight," the doctor warned. "He's nervous!"

This time, a woman technician took John's X-rays. Afterward, she invited us in to wait with John for the results. John, intrigued with the X-ray equipment, chatted calmly. He was more confident in our presence. An aide told us later that the X-ray department had a new policy. Parents were being encouraged to accompany their children for X-rays.

Back in John's room later that morning, the head nurse delivered a message to us from Dr. Morello. "The gall bladder X-rays were all right. The gall bladder was not touching the stomach after all." John vomited the tranquilizers. He then said he thought he felt better. We relaxed a bit, and Jack returned to work.

But in just a short time, out in the hall, a nurse gave me another message from Dr. Morello. She said softly, "Dr. Morello said to tell you that you can go back to St. Luke's." The anger in me flared again. He knew we had no choice but to stay! St. Luke's had no cobalt machine.

I tried to shrug it off, saying, "I really don't think John is able." Looking through the open door, I studied the boy in the bed, a boy who was fighting a malignant tumor of the spinal cord and desperately in need of radiation. I re-entered his room and made my way over to the window. Slumping down in the armchair, I silently stared out at the clouds. *Dear God, please help us!*

But John, still on tranquilizers under Dr. Morello's orders, continued to vomit. Two nights later, the nurses, unable to stand it any longer, again urged us to talk to the doctor. Although Jack loathed the thought of another confrontation, that night he approached the doctor out in the hall and said, "I think we'd better take the boy off tranquilizers, Dr. Morello. They certainly aren't helping him. Let's just take him off them and see what happens."

"All right," Dr. Morello said.

The next day, John rallied. As his spirits improved, he was able to get through the remainder of the radiation treatments without medication. And the prayers continued.

Curious Circumstances

Later in December on a bright afternoon, my neighbor, Betty Jackson, and I walked into the hospital. The crisp snow on the sidewalk crunched under our boots. Her son, Tom, was one of John's close friends. When we entered John's room, we walked past a thin, dark-haired woman in her fifties who sat crying by the empty bed near the door. We said nothing. I had not met John's new roommate, although for the past two days he had been a patient in that bed.

After we had visited with John for a moment, the woman burst out, "They moved my husband to Westminster Hospital today without my even knowing it." Burying her face in her hands, she sobbed into a white handkerchief. Westminster was thirty miles away.

"Why did they do that?" we asked softly.

"I don't know. Westminster is closer to our home. That's all I know," she cried.

"And they didn't tell you that they were moving him?" It seemed hard to believe, and we stared at her questioningly. "Perhaps it's a misunderstanding," I said, trying to placate her.

Shaking her head vigorously, she told us about the paralysis on the left side of her husband's body. I had noticed the day before when they brought him in from the recovery room that his left arm was in a sling and that he did not move in the bed. That afternoon, John had complained that the man had groaned several times the previous night and called out repeatedly, "Oh my God, my God, I can't believe it!"

Distraught and alone, the woman cried out, "What do you think I should do?"

"Who's your doctor?" I asked.

"Dr. Morello," she replied, wiping her eyes with the handkerchief. Her husband had never been sick before, and she had just learned of his paralysis.

"Why don't you pray?" I said. It was the only answer I could give her.

"Do you really think prayers help?" she cried.

"I know they do," I answered.

When Betty and I headed for the cafeteria later, the woman followed us out into the hall. "Good luck!" we called out after her, and then moved on, back to our own problems.

***

Three months later, the telephone rang in my husband's office. I answered.

"Is Jack there?" a male voice inquired.

"No," I replied. "Could I take a message?"

"This is Mr. Johnson," the voice continued.

"Who?" I tried to think of a customer by that name in our electrical business.

"Johnson. George Johnson. Don't you remember? I was in the hospital with your son."

"Which hospital?" I asked. John had been in three hospitals, with many different roommates.

"Benjamin Taylor," he replied. "I wasn't there very long. They moved me to Westminster Hospital because of the paralysis on my one side."

"Yes, oh yes," I said, recalling the details that his wife had told me. "Your wife was very upset. Did they really move you to Westminster Hospital without her knowing it?" Apparently she had told him about her conversation with Betty and me.

"Yessir," he asserted, "they did. They didn't even tell me. I was eating lunch that day when the ambulance men came in and said, 'Come on, you're going!' That was the first I knew of it. I didn't even have time to finish eating."

"Unbelievable!" I said. "How come they did that?"

"I don't know. I never asked. I wasn't able. I was very sick at the time."

Silence. Then, breaking the pause with hearty laughter, he continued, "But I'm feeling good now. The good Lord came through. I had my right eye removed last year. There was a malignancy there. Apparently they didn't get all of it, and it went to my brain. After they did tests in Westminster, they sent me to Rockleigh. They gave me some new kind of treatment up there. They thought I would lose my memory, but I didn't. The doctor said he might write me up in a medical journal. Some accomplishment, eh?" he said, laughing again.

Silence.

"I can walk with a cane now," he went on cheerfully.

"You can!" I marveled. Then I asked, "And you think the good Lord came through?"

"Think it? I *know* it! I'm positive of it." After a pause, he repeated, "Do I think the good Lord came through? That I recovered at all was nothing short of a miracle!"

After I had filled Mr. Johnson in on what was happening with John, I hung up the phone, feeling renewed. Hearing the good news gave me added strength to continue. Sometimes I felt so alone in the battles I was facing....

CHRISTMAS AND THE SPIRIT

One night during Advent, I picked up the local newspaper and scanned a story written by Gordon Hanson, an Associated Press writer. When I noticed the striking similarity between his story and ours, I hurried on to the ending, only to learn that his son had died. I then carefully reread the entire story:

FOUND PEACE IN SPIRIT THAT CAME AT CHRISTMAS[6]

EDITOR'S NOTE: Christmas is a time of joy, but it comes in the midst of realities that also include suffering, just as it did with Jesus, whose life from the first confronted hardship, exile, danger, eventually death and triumph over it. The following story involves the writer's family, which also faced distress but found an answer to it in the light of the life that came at Christmas.

Pain was Billy's ever-present companion. It delayed his falling asleep at night. It was with him through the long, dark hours, and it was his first wakening awareness every morning.

For the last two of Billy's 11 young years, the pain had shadowed him. He grew thinner. His cheeks were drawn and his eyes haunted.

Billy's pain was the terrible aftermath of a tobogganing accident. He had been flipped from the rear of one toboggan, and as he was sitting in the snow another toboggan came from behind and struck him in

[6] Associated Press, December 20, 1971.

the back. A tumor developed on his spine, and though his parents were unaware, it was turning cancerous.

Desperately Billy's parents sought a cure. Billy was their only child. There could be no more.

They took the boy from doctor to doctor, hoping one would say, 'I think I can help him.' But never was there any encouragement.

The search didn't end until the day a wizened, aging doctor in a small town far from Billy's home examined the boy.

"Bill will soon be free of pain," he said. "Soon he'll know it no longer."

Billy's mother knew that soon Billy would die.

But his father refused that interpretation. In his grief he accepted only that Billy would live. He needed that belief—that faith—to keep going. He couldn't let the boy down. The lad needed his strength, and he needed his son's.

The week before Christmas, Billy's fever rose. His pain worsened and only constant medication brought token relief.

The father raged in his anguish. He ranted to [sic] the futility of it all...the cruelty of God and the pointlessness of taking a life so young. Everything was a lie.

He knew no solace.

Then came Christmas Eve. The father was awakened by the sounds of Billy tossing fitfully in his bed.

Walking into the darkened living room, the father looked at the presents under the tree.

There were so many unopened gifts there for Billy. They represented the plans so carefully made for the boy.

The father slumped into a chair. He put his hands to his face and he wept.

Then, when grief could no longer come, he sat still for long minutes. The clock on the mantle [sic] ticked silently. He searched into himself, painfully and with determination.

And he remembered.

Slowly, awkwardly, he got down on his knees. Clasping his hands until the knuckles whitened, he raised his head.

"God," he said in an anguished whisper, "something has happened. I ask that you hear me out.

As I sat here, I remembered what a personal success I've been, and how you've responded when I asked you to give me a hand.

But I know now that these were selfish prayers, for my own personal gain. And when I asked you to save Billy, that was personal too.

I couldn't stand to lose him. I had such great plans for him and I wanted some day for him to carry on for me.

You know what I remember now? I remember your Son and Your great love when You gave Him to the world. What sadness You must have known when He died. And so, God, if you would do this great thing for all of us, then I must be comforted by Your sacrifice.

It's long past the time, oh God, when I must put my trust in You. So I pray that You will welcome little Billy when he comes. I know he'll be in good hands. I know that it is thy will be done."

The father got to his feet and went into Billy's bedroom. It was time for a pill.

The boy lay still. It almost seemed he wasn't breathing. On his cheek was a dried tear brought by the pain of only minutes before.

Tenderly the father took Billy's limp hand. He looked upon the boy he loved. Suddenly the little hand tightened. Billy opened his eyes.

"Dad," he said simply, "I won't be needing that pill tonight!"

Desperately, the father closed his eyes. Then he took a deep breath and asked the question he knew he must.

"Why not, Billy?"

"I've been dreaming, Dad. I've been dreaming about Jesus. He seemed very close. It might sound funny, but it's almost like He's here in the room with us right now."

Billy's fingers loosened in his father's grasp. The breath of life so silent it could barely be heard escaped his lips in a sigh. And his eyes closed.

The father bent over little Billy, and he took the tiny hands and folded them.

Straightening, he quietly spoke his final words to his son. "That wasn't a dream, Billy. And what you said about it probably sounding silly—it didn't.

He's here and He's watching over you...and me. He's watching over both of us.

Goodby [sic], son."

As I read this father's story, I found myself crying out to him, "Oh, God, no!" I wondered how he could bear it. However, I knew that our ending would be different. Our son would live.

THE 10,000TH PATIENT

Just after the New Year, we walked down the hall of Benjamin Taylor to freedom—freedom from cobalt treatments—for the present, at least. As a young blonde nurse pushed John in the wheelchair toward an open door, she told him, "I just finished filling in the charts, John. You're our 10,000th patient!"

"In how long a period?" I interjected.

"Three years," she replied.

John's eyes brightened. "I am? Then what do I get for a prize? A Jaguar? A ticket to Paris?"

"Gee, that's right, John," the nurse said, gazing at the floor thoughtfully. "You ought to get something."

"How about a one-way ticket out of here?" I suggested. "Wouldn't that be sufficient?" Then, becoming enthusiastic at the prospect, I gave John's chair a shove, adding, "Come on—John, let's—get—out of here!" John sped ahead of us down the hall in the wheelchair.

Then, turning to the nurses in the hallway, I said, "Thanks, gals, for everything. You've been wonderful!"

"Mrs. Redmond?" I heard a voice call after me.

"Yes?" Turning around, I saw Dr. Rodriguez coming toward us.

"He shouldn't have any trouble when he goes home, but if he does, call me. I'm here every afternoon."

"All right," I said happily. "And Dr. Rodriguez—thanks for everything you've done. Your department has been wonderful."

His eyes lit up. "Oh, we like to think so, Mrs. Redmond," he said. Stepping closer to us, he added confidentially, "You know, we not only have a hookup with Rockleigh, but we also have connections with St. Jude Children's Hospital in Memphis."

He paused, then continued, "You know—that's Danny Thomas's hospital." He searched my eyes, wondering if I knew the story.

"Yes, I know," I nodded, smiling. "I've read about it." And I thought about Danny Thomas, unemployed, in desperate need, praying to St. Jude for a job. He promised St. Jude that if he answered his prayers, he would donate some money to a charity in his honor. When St. Jude came through, Danny, with the help of others, founded a hospital dedicated to cancer research—the St. Jude Children's Research Hospital. His donations, along with millions of others, had funded research that offered new hope to cancer patients everywhere.

I left the department of radiology with a new respect for medical technology. Although John's care at Benjamin Taylor had been decidedly uneven, the radiologists had indeed been compassionate and helpful. For all the rest that had happened, I blocked it out of my mind. I could not dwell on the past. We had to move forward.

Dr. Morello would discharge John that weekend, almost six weeks after he was admitted to Benjamin Taylor.

Going Home

When we entered his room on Thursday afternoon, John greeted us with "Dr. Morello discharged me today."

"He did? How come?" I had thought he was going to discharge John on the weekend.

"So I can go home tomorrow."

"What did he say? Anything?"

"No, just that he's sending my papers up to Dr. Ferreira so he will know the case."

Earlier in the week, Dr. Morello had mentioned to me that John should go back to Cobourg Hospital for physical therapy under Dr. Ferreira's supervision. Although I dared not mention it to him, I had asked Dr. Hofmann while we were at St. Luke's if we could bring John back there for rehabilitation. Their rehab center was rated one of the finest of the few in the state.

"Should he go to an orthopedic surgeon now for physical therapy?" I had asked Dr. Morello.

"Yes," he replied.

"Well, then, I guess that's all right," I said, not wanting to anger him.

Later, I queried John. "Did Dr. Morello tell you to make an appointment with him for a checkup after you're out of the hospital?"

John shook his head. "No, he didn't say anything about that at all."

"Hmm. That's funny. It seems as if you ought to be checked by someone."

The next afternoon, I went down to the desk and requested a favor from the receptionist. "If a priest comes in," I said, "would you ask him to come up to our room? We're taking my son home today, and I'd like him to have the priest's blessing before he rides home in the car." I was worried about possible damage to John's spinal cord.

The receptionist seemed doubtful. "W-w-well, I will if one of them comes in," she replied, "but there hasn't been a priest in this hospital all week."

Feeling optimistic, I insisted, "Well, ask one if he comes in, will you?"

But the receptionist was right. No priests showed up that day. Still, we were happy to get out of the hospital and take our son home.

***

The following week, we received from Dr. Morello a surgical bill for $750. It came with the following notification: "This bill is due and payable at once. Dr. Morello is not a participating physician in Blue Shield." In 1971, the purchase price of a new car—a four-door Datsun 1200, for instance—was $2,100. By that standard, $750 was a huge amount of money.

Since Jack was self-employed, we had to pay the entire premium on our health insurance. We had counted on our Blue Shield insurance to cover the cost of the surgery, but the company honored bills only from participating physicians. It was shocking to learn, therefore, that John's surgery was not covered.

Dr. Hofmann had not yet submitted his bill, even though eight weeks had passed since our last visit with him. He had presided over a five-hour operation during which he had removed four vertebrae and a malignant tumor on the spinal cord. In addition, during his rounds, he had stopped in to see John several times even after he was no longer the attending physician in the case. We wondered what *his* bill would be like! After seeing what Dr. Morello was charging, we were very apprehensive.

Finally, one sunny afternoon when the bare branches of the trees in our yard had formed intricate patterns of shadows on the glistening snow, I went out to get the mail. As I opened the mailbox, I saw that the wind had blown the snow through the cracks around the door, and the mail was damp. Dr. Hofmann's bill was on the top of the stack of letters. With shivering hands, I ripped open the envelope, bracing myself for the shock.

But when I looked at the bill these words came to my mind: *By their fruits ye shall know them.* It read:

For professional services:

Neur. cons. and exam at request of Dr. Ferreira	$ 35.00
Myelogram	75.00
Hospital visits (2)	14.00
	$124.00
From Blue Shield	85.00
	$ 39.00 bal.

I immediately wrote Dr. Hofmann a note expressing my appreciation for his kindness. The man who had the right to charge more had charged less. And I was very grateful.

Brave Warriors

Four weeks after leaving the hospital, we took John back to Dr. Rodriguez for a checkup. When the doctor asked me if a neurosurgeon would also examine my son, I replied that Dr. Morello had neither transferred John to another neurosurgeon nor asked us to make another appointment with him.

Aware of our continuing conflicts with Dr. Morello, Dr. Rodriguez suggested, "Why don't you go to Dr. Hofmann?"

I hesitated, not knowing if this would meet with Dr. Hofmann's approval. But Dr. Rodriguez was insistent. "Dr. Hofmann would like to see him," he said.

We took John to see Dr. Hofmann one week later. That evening, Lynn, John, and Christopher bantered in their usual manner around the dinner table. Finally, Jack turned the conversation to John's checkup that morning.

Looking toward John, he said, "I asked Dr. Hofmann today about the size of the tumor that he removed from your spine, and he showed me one-third of his little finger."

John, the science buff, quickly shot back, "What are tumors made of?"

"Matter—and disorderly cells," Jack answered.

"Oh, that's cancer, not a tumor," Lynn interjected, chewing on a carrot as she brushed her long hair back over her shoulder.

John's face sobered, and an awkward silence fell around the table.

I glared at Lynn, and underlining each word carefully, I said, "*He had a tumor!*" She was aware of the nature of John's illness, and she also knew that he had not been told about it.

Unruffled, Lynn looked at John through narrowed eyes and put on a cold, expressionless face. Addressing him by the nickname known only to our children, she took another bite from the carrot and said, "You've got cancer, Dude. You've got only one month to live!" Holding her sides, she laughed uproariously.

Christopher, who also knew the truth about John's illness, quickly picked up on the cover-up. Giggling, he chimed in, "Yeah, Dude. You're gonna die!"

The mirth was contagious, and John thrust a fist upward, shouting, "Yeah! The sole survivor of cancer!" The whole idea seemed so ridiculous to him that he joined the others in hilarious laughter.

Physical Therapy

To the newcomer, the department was a whir of wheels with handles and ropes, pulleys and weights, and mirrors reflecting limp bodies lined up for renovation. Along the far wall were steel walkers arranged neatly in a row, and leaning against the wall were wooden crutches. Ashen-faced stroke victims slouched in wheelchairs, awaiting their turn to be lifted to the parallel bars, where two nurses held them while they straightened their legs. A third nurse stood in attendance with a wheelchair in case a patient felt faint.

Therapists teased Anne, a stroke victim in her fifties, by asking her how she was doing. Hard as they tried to inveigle a "Good" out of her, with brown eyes twinkling, she always replied, "Fair." She was destined to remain in a wheelchair, and she had told her sister that she would rather die than accept that fate.

Two accident victims, a boy and a girl in their early teens, with plaster casts on their fractured legs, winced in pain as they stood up for the first time and the blood rushed to their toes. Balancing themselves shakily, they straightened their bodies and learned to use their crutches. After a few days, when they had regained some strength, they practiced climbing stairs, with the nurses chanting, "Up with the good leg, down with the bad."

Frank, in gray chino trousers and a red plaid cotton shirt, pulled weights three times a week to strengthen the muscles in his once fractured shoulder. When his muscles convulsed as he lay on the exercise mat on the bed, he writhed in pain and begged the attendants to let him stop.

The twenty-six-year-old muscular Adonis in the wheelchair was a millionaire—the sole beneficiary of his parents' accident insurance policy following their death in a plane crash. He had fallen at his home, where he lived alone, and he had lain at the foot of the stairs for nineteen hours before someone found him. He insisted that he would walk and go scuba diving again.

Still tanned from the Caribbean sun, he flexed his powerful biceps as he propelled his wheelchair. Drawing himself up to his full six-foot height on the parallel bars, he gazed down at his tanned, lifeless legs and ordered them to walk. They did, day by day, an inch at a time, until he was able to walk home.

Old Mr. Newton came to soak his legs in the warm water of the whirlpool and to ride the bicycle-like contraption that was attached to a chair. After he had finished, he would stand over John, who lay almost lifeless on an exercise mat, and scold, "You do your exercises, young man!" Apparently, one of the therapists had told him that John was reluctant to exercise and that he would move only when someone moved him.

The old man went on, "When my son was your age, he had polio. He had to do exercises for a year, but his exercises pulled him through."

"Is he all right now?" I asked.

"Yes, he's married and has three children. He's a guidance counselor here in a Cobourg school." Choking back tears, he continued, "At first he was going to be a lawyer, then he ran a computer for a while, but he didn't have the strength to do it."

Then, turning to John again, he admonished, "You do your exercises, young man—you hear? It will make a difference for the rest of your life!" Then, with soulful eyes, he said to me, "Just keep your faith. It will pull you and him through."

The most remarkable thing about physical therapy was the humor and high spirits that we found there. Those who had the most to cry about were laughing instead. Although they were mostly helpless, they liked to pretend that they were independent. They also liked to tease the head of physical therapy, Maggie Foster, a lean, six-foot tall woman in her early fifties. Dressed in her white uniform and white oxfords, Maggie accepted all the ribbing good-naturedly as she carefully supervised her patients' activities.

When she gave John a command to do something, John, chuckling, would reply, "I won't."

Smiling, she would reply, "John, I used to be a captain in the Army. Now lift your leg as I say! I'll get my captain's bars out if you don't!" Every wheelchair victim in the room would laugh, egging him on to defy her.

She was the strength they lacked. "I'm tired today. I don't feel like it," John would complain, until she tossed a pillow at him to get him moving. The one thing her patients didn't want from her was pity.

But being a patient in physical therapy could be hazardous, too. After reviewing John's case history on our first visit, Mrs. Foster pointed out that John, under the direction of a physical therapist, had moved about with the aid of a walker at Benjamin Taylor. Tactfully implying that a good physical therapist would not have put a patient such as John on his feet immediately, she explained that, by prescribing the wrong exercises, an incompetent therapist could destroy a back surgery patient who had been bedridden for six weeks.

Once again we learned that we had skirted the edge of a cliff unawares, with only our guardian angels to pull us out of danger. But I did not believe in guardian angels.

***

John, who now weighed just 89 pounds, finally settled down to an exercise program of two hours daily for three months. Although his body was lifeless, he still had a twinkle in his eye when Jack or Rob carried him to the car each day to go to the hospital. At the emergency entrance, an aide took him in a wheelchair to Rehabilitation. There John was lifted to the exercise mat on a king-size hospital bed.

Slowly, a transformation took place. It seemed as if we were watching a miracle when we saw John lift his right leg, pull his arms and head up a little, or move his hips just a bit to one side. "Oh, boy! I could do this all day!" he would exclaim as he swung his five-foot, six-inch body down through the parallel bars, moving one leg feebly after the other. The other patients cheered him on while an aide stood beside him to catch him if he faltered.

Then, from across the room, Maggie Foster would yell, "Come on, John, that's enough for today! Don't overdo it!"

"Oh, boy!" he'd say again, seeming not to hear her. He was like a baby taking his first steps. And, like a one-year-old, exhilarated by his new-found power, he'd wobble on, moving one leg slowly after the other.

"Come on, John, that's enough!" Mrs. Foster would call again. His eyes passionate now, John would repeat, "Oh, boy! I could do this all day!"

I looked away with tears of thanks in my eyes. I felt so humble. Oh, God can be good!

After three months on a schedule as rigorous as that of an Olympic trainer, John began exercising at home, using pulleys, weights, and an exercise bike. He returned to physical therapy twice a week so that Mrs. Foster could check on his progress.

He now walked with Lofstrand crutches that fit around the arm, below the elbow, with a curved strip of metal. The rubber-padded bars at hand-level enabled him to support himself. He was grateful to be spared the cumbersome wooden crutches that fit under the armpit. Inside our home, he could walk by himself for a short distance without any support.

This was the awakening we'd dreamed of—the end of that dreadful nightmare.

Beyond a Fifth-Grade Education

God gave us Life to seek Him;
Death to find Him;
Eternity to possess Him.

-Author unknown

Throughout this time of suffering, Christopher gained wisdom. In the large bedroom that he and John had shared, instead of the usual boys' clutter, everything was in its place. Christopher lacked the heart to play without John there.

Yet our son did find out who answers prayers. Although he always petitioned with the loudest voice around the dinner table, *Hail Mary, full of grace, the Lord is with thee...*I never realized the intensity of his feelings until three months after John came home from the hospital. While cleaning off the kitchen counter one morning, I picked up a lined sheet of white paper and scanned it to see if I should toss it into the wastebasket. When I saw that it was Christopher's homework, I reread it more carefully. It said:

Cobourg County Airport
Airport Road

Gentlemen:

Please tell me when my fifth grade class attending CCS could come on a tour. We would like to go on an airliner that you have.

I have Forty pupils in the class. I would like to bring them at one o'clock.

Sincerely yours,

Christopher Redmond

On the other side of the paper, he had written:

O Dear God I thank you for
making my brother well.
he is feeling very good. Thank you
Dear God

It was another confirmation that, in order to become wiser, we sometimes have to experience suffering.

HITCHHIKING 101

Although we came together as a family every night around the dinner table, we were each on our own as to how to cope with John's illness. Rob's way was to get out of town. One evening, Jack told me that after John and I had left the house that morning to go to physical therapy, Rob apprised him—as he was going out the door—that he was leaving for the Bahamas.

"The Bahamas!" I repeated incredulously. "How did he go?" He had no means of transportation.

"They're going to hitchhike," Jack answered. Rob was traveling with a classmate, Mark Williams, whom we knew well.

The politics of the times had polarized families, friends, and neighbors. In 1996 Walter Cronkite referred to the 1960s as "the most turbulent decade of the century," adding that this was the most difficult period in which to raise children in the nation's history.[7]

During our discussions around the dinner table, Rob had often said that this polarization was due to a lack of communication. He explained that one of the reasons he liked to hitchhike was so that he and the driver could visit and get to know each other, thereby promoting tolerance. Although we agreed with his philosophy, we warned him that his method of practicing it was risky. But Rob hitchhiked anyway.

Neither Jack nor I tried to stop Rob the day he left for the Bahamas. We knew our efforts would be fruitless. It was the beginning of spring break, and by the time we finished talking about his plans, he had already left town. I

---

7 "Cronkite Remembers," CBS documentary using archival footage and home movies to illustrate a newsman's unique perspective on history, May 23, 1996.

sighed, shrugged, and went to bed, knowing that I had to muster up enough strength to take John to physical therapy the next day. Jack, tired from daily physical work, settled down in his recliner to read the paper.

At the end of the following week, Rob returned. Relieved that he was unharmed, I asked, "How was it?" I had always dreamed of going to the Bahamas.

"OK," he assured me.

"How much money did you have with you?" I asked. I couldn't comprehend how he had scraped up enough money to go to the Bahamas. His job as a dishwasher at the airport restaurant paid minimum wage.

"Thirty-five dollars," he replied matter-of-factly.

"Thirty-five dollars!" I repeated, horrified.

"No, Mom, it was OK," he said. "People were just wonderful to us. We made out just fine!"

"Like how?" I asked, still disbelieving.

"Well, it was raining one night when we were hitchhiking, and this guy picked us up in a station wagon. When he let us out, he insisted that I take his poncho to keep dry. He said that Mark and I could trade off with it. Everybody was great to us, really."

Shaking my head, I repeated, "Thirty-five dollars! How did you eat?"

"Oh, in one place we sat at the counter in a diner and ordered coffee. This older guy sat next to us and must have overheard us talking about how hungry we were. He told us to order two dinners and he would pay for it. We couldn't believe it. People were so nice."

Jack, who had been listening quietly, finally spoke up.

"How old was this guy?" he asked.

"Oh, I dunno," Rob said, shrugging his shoulders. "Probably in his late forties, early fifties."

Jack chuckled. "Oh, I see who was responsible for your wonderful time—two guys forty-five or fifty, one driving a station wagon. Sounds like the Establishment to me." He was alluding to "Down with the Establishment," a popular slogan of the time, especially among college students.

"The very people you guys criticize were the ones most generous and thoughtful toward you!" Jack teased. "How do you explain that?"

Rob had no explanation. He just reaffirmed his belief in the goodness of mankind.

***

That same year, Rob learned about the dark side of hitchhiking. While thumbing a ride home from work one night, two drunks picked him up in a two-door Volkswagen and refused to let him out. Laughing merrily, they passed a liquor bottle back and forth as they drove on past Cobourg with Rob in the back seat.

Jack listened quietly while Rob recounted the story, but Lynn, John, Christopher and I asked, "What did you do, Rob, when they wouldn't let you out?"

"Oh, nothing," Rob replied casually. "I wasn't going to play games with those jerks. I just put my head back and went to sleep!"

"Went to sleep!" we exclaimed. "Weren't you too scared to?"

Rob's eyes widened. He laughed and shook his head. "Well, yeah, I was, but what could I do?" he replied. "I wasn't going to give those guys the satisfaction of knowing that they were scaring the heck out of me!"

During the four or five hours in which Rob was feigning sleep, the two men had driven into a neighboring state. Finally, at 2:30 a.m., they pulled over to the curb along a deserted street and let Rob out.

Relieved, Rob had located a YMCA that provided rooms for travelers. There, after he had related his story, the night clerk lent him $15 to cover the cost of a room, securing from Rob a pledge that he would repay the loan as soon as he got home. His faith in mankind restored, Rob happily put $15 in an envelope the next morning and sent it off to the good Samaritan. However, his interest in hitchhiking waned considerably after that incident.

John's blue eyes danced as he listened to Rob's escapades. Although he was basically a shut-in, hobbling around on crutches, the adrenaline flowed. Hardly able to contain himself, he snickered through most of the story every time he repeated it to one of his visiting friends. Living dangerously through his brother was a good dose of medicine for him.

THE FLOOD

At 4:30 a.m. in May of 1972, a nightmarish lady named Hurricane Angie ripped through Cobourg without any warning. In just one half-hour, she wiped out twenty lives and hurled the belongings of thousands of city residents into the street. There they sat—a water-drenched mess oozing mud.

Only thirty minutes earlier sandbagged dikes surrounding the city had broken in seven places. Voices blaring from police car bullhorns urged unsuspecting city dwellers to evacuate their homes immediately. Sleepy residents telephoned their neighbors, grabbed a few belongings, and scurried for their lives as the ten-foot wall of water swept through the community. Communications were cut off, families were separated, and life in Cobourg ground to a standstill.

While a handful of stunned local officials and the National Guard struggled to bring order out of chaos, men, women, and children huddled together in evacuation centers or in homes outside the area and swapped horror stories, recounting their experiences during that dreadful night.

Maynard Jackson, an old man who had the use of only one arm and one leg after suffering a stroke, limped around with a crutch and a cane. After he and his wife separated, he lived in the upstairs apartment of their home, and she lived downstairs.

Several days before the flood, it had rained relentlessly. Police officers repeatedly checked the depth of the river with gauges, but according to radio reports that night, there was no cause for alarm. The river would crest within hours, we were assured. However, Maynard felt uneasy, and around 3:30 a.m., he telephoned downstairs to his wife.

"Mary," he fretted. "That river's rising. Let's get out of here while there's still time!"

But furious that he had awakened her, Mary snapped back, "Listen, you fool, if you ever call me again in the middle of the night and wake me up, I'll—I'll kill you!" With that, she slammed the receiver down.

Maynard had no choice but to wait. With a gnawing uneasiness, he peered out the window repeatedly, watching the rising commotion in the street below. By 4 a.m., when the sirens sounded and the bullhorns blared directions to evacuate, Maynard had planned his course of action.

Hobbling out from the living room with his crutch and cane, he hoisted himself into the kitchen sink. When the huge wall of water slammed past his house, he huddled in the sink with his head between his legs, spitting the water out of his mouth.

Suddenly, a savior appeared at the kitchen window—a man in white boxer shorts who had been swept down by the waters from his apartment two blocks away. As he grabbed hold of Maynard's window, much to his surprise, he stopped. When the waters subsided, the involuntary hero half-carried, half-dragged Maynard out to the roof, where they waited for rescuers in boats to pick them up.

Although some took precautionary measures, others did nothing. Nancy Denson, a forty-year-old woman living alone in a two-story apartment building in the neighboring town of Fairfield, slept peacefully while the building's other 300 occupants telephoned one another frantically, sounding the alarm to evacuate.

Because Nancy traveled frequently in her job, no one knew that she was home until she was awakened at 7 a.m. by a man's voice yelling, "Hal-lo? Anybody there?" The rescuer had returned in an amphibious vehicle to check on a dog he'd heard barking at 4:15 a.m. when he drove away with the other apartment evacuees.

Nancy, sleepily pulling on her robe, ambled out to the balcony. Recognizing the man outside, she yelled, "Hey, Fred, what's goin' on? I've gotta be at the airport this morning at nine o'clo—," but her voice trailed off as she looked around her. Fred was in a boat in water that was almost up to the second-floor landing where she stood! It took a little time for

Nancy to grasp the situation, but she'd managed to get a good night's sleep while her neighbors were scrambling for their lives.

An exhausted waitress living alone on the Northside returned home on the eve of the flood after working eight hours. She ate a sandwich, then went upstairs to bed. While sirens screeched and bullhorns blared, she slept on, and when she awoke, she was floating in water an arm's length away from the ceiling. Edging herself over to a window, she got out onto the roof, where she clung to a television cable until a man in a boat rescued her.

A few days after Angie had passed through, a man resembling Yul Brynner scrawled a question in white paint on the side of his devastated house: "WHERE THE HELL IS THE GREAT WHITE KNIGHT WHEN YOU NEED HIM?"

Within a few weeks, those words, written in jest, had boomeranged. A photographer announced that in one of his black-and-white prints of the disaster he thought he saw a white-robed figure—a white, bearded male—with arms outstretched, hovering above the destruction, with the sleeves of his loose garment hanging freely against his sides.

As the picture circulated, many agreed that they could see the figure of Jesus Christ in the print. Others could not see it at all. And the question arose: Was the Great White Knight really there? When school began in the fall, students passed copies of the print around their classrooms. Some students agreed that they, too, could see Christ in the sky, spreading protective arms over the damaged city.

After three weeks of backbreaking work shoveling mud and collecting waterlogged debris, a muscular volunteer in his twenties expressed his sentiments in just one word. He wore a smile button turned upside down on his faded blue T-shirt, making the smile a frown, with a tongue hanging out. And below the face he had written a word so descriptive of the muddy-brown substance that covered the city—"SHIT."

But as Cobourg slowly came back to life, a spirit of love, unity, and hope replaced the materialistic self-centeredness that had previously prevailed. A sign on the rolling green lawn of a farm equipment store in Hillsdale, a neighboring town, said it all. It commented dryly: "ANGIE WAS NO LADY."

Ups and Downs

In 1962, we sold our home in an area that would be heavily flooded ten years later, and we built a house on a hill three miles outside the city. At that time, we never dreamed that one June morning we would look out in awe from our kitchen window and see mobile homes floating in murky floodwaters in the valley below. Helicopters carrying rescuers circled our area continuously, looking for stranded residents. We watched as three persons clinging to a silo on a large dairy farm near us were pulled to safety.

At first, the only priority was survival. Some lacked shelter or food, and everyone was without electricity and water. In our home, our immediate concern was caring for a dependent teenager on crutches. Health officials warned that even in surrounding areas, residents should boil their water because of possible surface contamination. But we had no electricity for our well pump or electric stove.

The road leading into Cobourg had been closed after Bedford Creek overflowed, and we had no contact with the devastated area for the first few days. On our street—a cul-de-sac with seven houses—only one neighbor was fortunate enough to have a transistor radio *and* batteries. From him we learned that the radio station nearby was broadcasting names of evacuees, trying to let their families know that they were alive.

Rob was one of the missing persons. He had been visiting his girlfriend, Beth, at her home in Cobourg on the eve of the flood. When he was ready to leave about 11 p.m., her parents, having heard radio reports that our bridge was out, convinced him to stay there with them. At 5 a.m., they had to evacuate to a nearby school, where they stayed the rest of the night. The next afternoon, they left the city on one of the few roads that was open, and they stayed with Beth's relatives in a neighboring town.

We did not have a transistor radio, so we never heard Rob's name mentioned in the list of evacuees. However, his two uncles, living 100 miles away in Stonehill, heard his name on the broadcast. I was convinced that Rob could take care of himself, and that wherever he was, he would be OK. He finally showed up on the third day.

Lynn and I spent most of our time preparing meals in the fireplace for the six of us, and we readily discovered that the toast we made for breakfast over the fire was the best we'd ever had. Fortunately, in nearby Canton, spring water flowed out of a pipe on private property, and the word spread quickly that the landowner had offered it for all to use freely. Men and boys stacked wood for the fireplaces and brought buckets of water from the spring for drinking, sponge bathing, washing dishes, and flushing toilets.

In the emergency areas, damage was in the multi-millions, and when 1,000 National Guardsmen arrived to protect the city against looters, the mayor imposed an 8 p.m. curfew for everyone.

The second day, Jack circumvented the flooded area by taking a back road, and he drove his van to a hillside overlooking the city. When he came home, he insisted that I go with him the next day to see the devastation. "You just won't believe it!" he said. Until that time, knowing only that a wall of water had been loosed on the city when the dikes broke, my concerns had been closer to home.

When Jack and I drove to the hillside the next day and looked across the river, we saw destruction that was incomprehensible. The new one-story elementary school in our old neighborhood was immersed up to the rooftop in muddy water. On top of a pile of debris that had once been a McDonald's, the golden arches forming the "M" lay askew. Our old house had been twisted off its foundation, along with most of the others in that area. Heavy trucks lay on their side or upside down. Utility poles had fallen across the streets and huge trees had been uprooted. Cars were double-parked, not side by side, but piggyback.

Since many adults had not had bathtubs in their early years, they were familiar with sponge baths. But the younger family members in our neighborhood, although they insisted on dressing in faded, tattered clothes, were accustomed to showering and shampooing daily. By the third day, sponge baths were not enough.

When the news spread that the shower rooms in the nearby Canton elementary school were open to the public, Lynn and Christopher ran to the van outside, where Jack waited for them, and John on his crutches followed them. After they had helped John into the van, the four of them took off.

At first, I was reluctant to go. The showers, they said, were in an open room with no privacy. But after listening to them rave nonstop about how good it felt to be clean, I, too, began to yearn for fresh, warm water spraying down on me. Two days later, I ventured out during the lunch hour to shower and shampoo, and I was lucky. I was there all by myself!

The curfew brought everyone closer together. Every night, we sat by candlelight, playing cards and swapping stories about our daily experiences. Rob and scores of other high-school and college students, full of youthful vigor and good humor, pitched in to clean up the city. As they worked side by side with discouraged homeowners, asking nothing for their labors, the generation gap narrowed, and many of our youths experienced the satisfaction of being needed for the first time.

With no advance notice, the lights came on one night a week later. At the time, Jack and Christopher were down in the garage checking the electrical pumps, heaters, and motors. We had looked forward to this moment, and now, finally, we were being relieved of the added burden of primitive living.

The older members of the family were in high spirits, so no one noticed that Christopher was quiet the whole time. Suddenly, he surprised us by announcing, "Oh, darn. I liked it the way it was!"

In the second week, most of the men joined forces in the city to provide essential services where they were needed. Jack worked with the Central

Electric & Gas Company employees who were trying to restore electricity to the devastated areas.

In January of that year, we had paid a deposit on a cottage at the ocean for our annual two-week vacation, and our reserved weeks were rapidly approaching. After weighing the pros and cons of forfeiting the deposit, we decided that, for John's sake, I would drive to the ocean with the younger children, and Jack and Rob would stay behind to help the flood victims. Jack would come down later when he could get away. It would be much easier for me to manage there. At home, our well water still had to be boiled, even for laundry.

The following Saturday, Lynn and I shoved our dirty laundry into huge black plastic lawn bags and headed for an overcrowded laundromat east of the city. After packing the clean, folded clothes back into the plastic bags, Lynn, John, Christopher, and I headed for the seashore. At the end of that week, the lights came on in Cobourg, and Jack headed south in his van.

Reveling in our new-found freedom, we stretched out on the sandy shores, rejuvenating ourselves in the ocean breezes and nourishing sun. John, with his blond hair sun-bleached and his fair skin tanned, seemed stronger. He ably withstood the ocean waves slapping him as he slowly made his way along the beach on the Lofstrand crutches.

In the evenings, we browsed in little boutiques and antique shops in the touristy downtown. We were amazed at the five-and-dime stores with their variety of bathing suits, beach equipment, towels, and toys that were unavailable in our hometown. To wind up the evening, we often headed for an old-fashioned ice cream shop to relish a hot dog or hamburger, a hot fudge peanut butter sundae with whipped cream and nuts, or a pistachio ice cream cone.

On a few lazy afternoons, up at the end of the island, we watched the sea gulls and pelicans dive for food while we soaked up the salt air and absorbed the fishy smells. Near the lighthouse, fishermen sat on the dock, patiently reeling in their lines at every imagined tug, and the sound of waves smacking up against the sea wall lulled each of us into our own reverie.

The day we were leaving for home, our landlord and landlady, a pleasant, retired couple who lived in the apartment above us, inquired, "How was it?"

We laughed and said, almost in unison, "Oh, just heavenly!"

Flattered, but disbelieving (we had told them little about our ordeal), they said, "Oh, come on, it couldn't have been that good!"

But it had been. For us, it was the ecstasy after the agony.

***

Our joyfulness was short-lived, however. Upon our return, when we took John to Dr. Hofmann for an examination, he told us that John would need surgery again. A second tumor had developed on his spinal cord—in the same place as the one that had just been removed. Although we were devastated, we kept our composure. We wanted to keep John's spirits up. John, in turn, was reluctant to upset us again, so he calmly accepted the news.

Following this surgery, the prognosis was straightforward. John would spend the rest of his life in a wheelchair.

***

During this difficult time, I ran into Helen Kennedy one day in the hospital's cafeteria. Helen and her husband, Chuck, lived near us. I hadn't heard that Chuck had suffered a severe heart attack and was hospitalized, so I was surprised to see Helen there. Over coffee, we discussed the prognoses of the two patients.

With a big sigh, I recounted John's condition. "Well, it's up to God," I told Helen. "I just pray, 'Thy will be done.'" I didn't know if it would be better for John to die or to spend the rest of his life in a wheelchair.

Helen countered immediately. "Well, I don't pray that way!" she said indignantly. "I pray that Chuck will get better! I won't have it any other way!"

I wondered then why I wavered so. Perhaps I should be more assertive with my requests to God, as Helen was. Jack and Lynn had talked with John about the logistics of getting him to school in the van after he came home to stay, but John and I never discussed the possibility or the reality of his being paralyzed.

I couldn't accept it. I had always treaded water as I'd dealt with life's blows, but this news seemed to be more than I could bear. Having four children had been one of my life's goals, but now, touching bottom, I wanted to die. Only once did I voice this aloud, and that was to Dr. Hofmann. One night, when we were discussing John's prognosis, I told him that I wanted to die if John did. I didn't tell him that it frightened me to feel like this. Indeed, the scariest thing was that I didn't even want to live for the sake of my other children—whom I loved dearly!

I had always marveled that the fingers, toes, ears, and nose of each of our newborns were positioned perfectly. Certainly this was a miracle, and it had reinforced my hazy belief in the doctrine that there was a God.

But that image appeared to be shattered now. I didn't believe I could handle what lay ahead.

Fate or Coincidence?

Because John was pale and bedridden now, some afternoons I pushed him in the wheelchair through the hospital corridors or took him outside into the warm sunshine. As we walked around the gardens, a childhood memory haunted me.

I had been thirteen at the time. I rode with my mother in our Ford sedan to Middletown, a city five miles south of our farm, to do the daily shopping for our evening meal. Because my mother was "not dressed," which meant that she did not have on her navy blue silk crepe dress, pearl earrings, pearl necklace, and black patent leather high-heeled pumps, she pulled into a parking space and told me to run into the Mohican bakery and get a whipped cream cake and "not one thing more." She reached into her purse and then handed me a dollar bill and some nickels, dimes, and quarters.

I rarely ran errands for my mother. My sister, Sylvia, who was four years older than I, usually did all the important things. But she was not with us that day.

Eagerly I climbed out from the back seat onto the running board of the car. I was wearing my favorite apricot piqué dress with green and pink flowers embroidered across the yoke. As I jumped down to the pavement, a gust of wind swept street dust into my eyes, and I threw up my hands to protect them. When the dust cleared, I stepped onto the curb and skipped happily along, with my shingle-bobbed brown hair bouncing.

As I did so, my eyes fell on a crippled old man in a wheelchair. He was alone in front of the Olympic theater. Slowing to a halt, I stared at him, mesmerized. Then slowly, catlike, I moved toward him. He was rattling a little tin cup and crying out in a barely audible voice, "Pencils? Pencils?" But the people on the street hurried on by, preoccupied.

As I drew nearer the bent head and the unshaven face, the man lifted his head, and I saw that he was blind. I faltered as my heart welled up in pity. Again I heard him cry, "Give to the blind? Give to the blind?"

Opening my fist that held within it the silver coins that my mother had given me, I moved toward him. Reaching out gingerly, I dropped three or four coins into his cup. When he heard the coins rattle, he handed me two pencils. Taking them from him, I turned and ran swiftly toward the Mohican.

I returned to the car skipping, but when I crawled inside, my mother, amused, questioned me about my pity for the poor old man. In those days, there was little public awareness of the plight of the handicapped.

Since it was not common at that time for adults to take children's words or actions seriously unless they misbehaved, my mother often entertained our dinner guests—usually relatives—with the story. "She gave money to the crippled old man in the wheelchair who begs!" she'd laugh. Looking down at my plate, I sat quietly, listening.

But later, when I was alone, bewildered, I would wipe the tears from my eyes. What had I done wrong? I wondered. Why was it so funny?

Now many years later, I pondered fate and coincidence. Now my son was in a wheelchair! I could not shake the image of that little old man who had torn at my heart as he begged on the public square.

***

Not long after the surgery to remove the tumor, John developed a bedsore on his left buttock. Since bedsores are difficult to heal on a paralyzed patient, Dr. Hofmann called in Dr. Mitchell, a plastic surgeon, who performed surgery on the bedsore. Afterward, John lay face down in bed or on a gurney with his arms extended so he could wheel himself through the corridors.

To prevent a recurrence, aides hinted to me that I might want to bring percale sheets from home for John's bed. They pointed out that the harsh disinfectants used in the hospital laundry on their coarse white muslin sheets might cause more skin irritation. To avoid a mix-up, I took two new sets of light blue percale sheets to the hospital. At my request, Dr. Hofmann left orders for the caregivers to leave John's soiled sheets in his room so that I could take them home to be laundered. With changing shifts and staff turnover, however, the blue sheets disappeared within a few weeks, and no one knew of their whereabouts.

During this eight-week period of healing, as John made his way through the halls face down on a gurney, he developed a camaraderie with the staff. They believed that love was healing, and he, thriving under their nurturing, absorbed every bit of love they showered upon him.

He and Marcia, a diminutive licensed practical nurse, developed an especially close relationship. Marcia, in her late thirties, was a divorcée with a son who was six years younger than John. Off duty, she wore tight blue jeans and usually pulled back her long blonde hair into a ponytail. During the winter, when she frequently visited John at home, she pulled off her snowy boots at the front door and walked around our house barefoot.

Marcia rarely talked to me, but when I entered John's room at home or in the hospital, she was often bending over him. They held hands and gazed at each other in whispered conversation. It would then cross my mind that Marcia was taking my place with John. But I was in such a crisis of my own, I had little strength to give anyone. Therefore, I was grateful that John was flourishing under her loving support. Later, however, their close relationship would prove to be an obstacle in my path when I resumed my role as his mother.

FAMILY VISITORS

Without telling us where he was going, Rob left one morning to hitchhike the 150 miles to his grandmother's apartment in Middletown. My sister, Sylvia, having flown up from Florida, was visiting my mother there. When Rob told them about John's predicament, they were shocked, but they assured Rob that they were praying for his brother. The next day they drove down to visit John and brought Rob back with them.

My mother paled when she saw her paralyzed grandson. Sylvia and I greeted each other coolly, and after a few hours, they left to return to Middletown.

Three years earlier an incident concerning John had alienated my sister from me. Sylvia and I had not spoken to each other since that last time we'd vacationed together at the ocean with our families. John was thirteen years old then, Christopher was nine, and Sylvia's boys, Pete and Joey, were ten and nine, respectively.

Every year, the four cousins eagerly looked forward to spending their vacation together. Each of them chattered about it as the time approached. However, the last summer we met, Sylvia, consumed with jealousy over the boys, became unreasonable.

While the two of us were having coffee in her cottage one day, she said, "Barbara, I don't like John!"

"For gosh sakes, Sylvia. Why?" I inquired. Had something happened that I didn't know about? Had John been picking on one or both of her boys, who were younger? If so, I would punish him immediately.

Looking down at her shoes, Sylvia twisted her beautiful face into a pout and said, "Because my boys like him too much. All they talk about is John, John, John!"

This was his sin—that he loved her boys? I exhaled, relieved that I would not have to punish John.

In earlier years, Sylvia and I had openly expressed our happiness that our four older children—Rob and Lynn, and her Bob and Susan—got along well together. Didn't she now want this same harmony for our younger ones?

Although she was a generous person, Sylvia was also competitive. Always quick to protect her self-appointed position as leader of the pack, she would rage when gripped with possessiveness, or protest loudly at the slightest trace of independent thinking on our part.

Because I was almost four years younger than Sylvia, I had deferred to her my entire life. She was beautiful, and thus she had always held center stage. When we were young, strangers often stopped my mother on the street to admire Sylvia's fair skin, blonde hair, blue eyes, and dimples. "Isn't she lovely!" they'd gasp.

Then, looking at me, they'd inquire, "And is this your other daughter?" When my mother nodded affirmatively, they either stared at me without comment or said, "Oh," and continued up the street. I, the plain one, was always in Sylvia's shadow.

Nevertheless, content with my secondary role, I happily became Sylvia's follower. I, too, admired her beauty. When we were teen-agers, it was exciting to watch boys turn toward us and whistle, even though I knew it was Sylvia they were admiring.

I could never decide whether Sylvia looked like Lana Turner or Betty Grable, but sometimes she acted more like Bette Davis. Through the years, she often hurt me with her lies and selfishness. She never admitted wrongdoing, but I always quickly forgave her, just wanting to restore peace. The truth was that I needed her. Our neighbors' children were older and no longer lived at home. Thus, Sylvia and I had only each other for companionship.

So, when Sylvia told me that day at the ocean that she didn't like John, I chalked it up to jealousy and shrugged it off. Her unhappiness seemed pointless. John hadn't done anything wrong. I never dreamed that my sister would give further vent to her anger—until the last day of our vacation.

I left the beach early that afternoon and went back to my place to put a roast in the oven. It was my turn to get dinner. Sylvia stayed on the beach with the boys so they could finish building their sand castles. Although Sylvia and I rented separate cottages, we and our families often ate our evening meal together.

When Sylvia drove up to the cottage an hour later, John and Christopher jumped out of the car and ran in ahead of her. Minutes later, she stormed into the living room, followed by her boys. Walking directly over to John, she bent down, looked him in the eye, and snarled, "Someone has stolen my beach chair!"

Both John and Christopher drew back from her, intimidated. I wondered why she would accuse John. She knew I'd brought our new beach chairs from home that summer.

Sylvia had always valued material things far beyond their worth. Compared with our frugal existence, she and her husband, Dave, lived in luxury. Dave, a regional manager for Brunswick Airlines, made a high five-figure salary, with excellent benefits. Conversely, although we had done well over the past five years with our electrical contracting business, politics and recessions were now affecting our income. We had just moved into our new house with four young children, and we had worked hard to realize that goal. We also had to plan financially a year in advance for our vacations, so we treasured every minute of them.

When Sylvia went outside to rinse the children's wet bathing suits under the faucet, John whispered, "Mom, Aunt Sylvia's beach chair is in her car trunk. I saw her put it there before we came up from the ocean!" Innocently, he thought that Aunt Sylvia's outburst had sprung from a lapse of memory. I did not reply. I knew that her memory was as sharp as ever.

When she came back into the cottage, I said, "Let's look in your car trunk for the beach chair, Sylvia." She declined adamantly, insisting that it was not there.

Having had enough of her lies and accusations, I became just as insistent. "Give me the keys," I said. "I'll look." I reached out my hand, but she gripped the keys tightly and held them to her chest. Her eyes shifted from side to side as she pondered what to do next.

Now that I had confronted Sylvia, she had no alternative but to go with me. We went to the car together, and the children followed us. When Sylvia opened the trunk, I saw parts of the folded beach chair peeking out from beneath wet towels and sandals. Giving her a look of disgust, I turned away quickly and started back toward the cottage. I thought of how my sister had always gotten by on her looks, so that she had never had to account for her actions.

Although I said nothing, I knew in my heart that I was through playing games with Sylvia. I also knew well the effect a lie could have upon the innocent. It was like choking on food with no one to help you.

Throughout my early years, whenever I was wrongly accused, I wished that a great white knight would appear and straighten things out for me. But it never happened. In those times, it seemed the universal thinking was that, since things are not always as they appear, one should stay out of other people's arguments.

That thinking changed after a stranger murdered Kitty Genovese in 1964 in Queens, New York. Thirty-eight persons, awakened at 3 a.m. by her screams on the street below, watched from their open apartment windows as an assailant stabbed her, and they did nothing to help. One man yelled from a window, "Let that girl alone," and the attacker walked away. But shortly thereafter, he returned twice to stab her again. And, as before, witnesses watched but did nothing. Police maintained that the woman's life might have been saved if just one witness had called them.

Twenty years later, Stanley Milgram, a psychology professor from the City University of New York, cited this incident at a scholarly conference at Fordham University. He asked his audience, "If we need help, will those around us stand around and let us be destroyed or will they come to our aid? Are those other creatures out there to help us sustain our life and values, or are we individual flecks of dust just floating around in a vacuum?"[8]

This tragedy became a classic case of "apathy among bystanders."

At the ocean that night, with Jack at the head of the table, we broke bread and conversed, but with little enthusiasm. Jack had been fishing that day and knew nothing of the incident. After dinner, out of habit, Sylvia and I kissed each other on the cheek and said goodbye.

When I got home, however, I indirectly accused her in a letter. I wrote, "Sylvia, what will you profit if you gain the whole world and suffer the loss of your soul? God gave us a new commandment, Sylvia—to love one another! I can't take it any longer. Goodbye." Knowing that Sylvia always took it out on those who defied her, I neither signed the letter nor put a return address on the envelope. She knew my handwriting, and the envelope would be postmarked "Cobourg."

A week later, I received from Sylvia a letter penned in red ink. It was not customary to use red ink for personal correspondence, and she had never used it before in writing to me. In the letter, she accused John of having written her an extremely disrespectful message, and she said that he should apologize to her at once. She insisted that she had neither lied nor made accusations about anyone.

In reply, I told her that I, not John, had written the letter, and that I had not even spoken with John about the incident. (How could I explain any of this to a young child?) But the letter was returned to me unopened, with the word "REFUSED" stamped on the envelope.

Once again, Sylvia had opted for war instead of the peace that I longed for.

---

8 Michael Dorman, "Long Island. Our Story. The Killing of Kitty Genovese," http://www.lihistory.com/8/hs818a.htm.

Little did I know then that, in the inscrutable providence of God, Sylvia would later be used as an instrument of grace to bring peace to my heart forever.

The Vigilant Protector

On another weekend, Jack's sister, Carol, brought John's paternal grandmother down for the day so she could visit her grandson in the hospital. My mother-in-law was like a mother to me, and my sister-in-law and I had always had a good relationship.

Although Jack and I had often talked on the phone with his parents, we had not seen them in two years. Jack's father, who was in his late seventies, had been intermittently ill and was not able to drive any distance. Thus, no one had told us that my mother-in-law had hardening of the arteries, which causes memory loss and changed behavior.

So on that particular Sunday afternoon, an incident occurred that caught me totally off guard. When we entered John's room, I was shocked to hear my mother-in-law let out a hearty, deep-throated laugh as she walked over to John's bed and saw him lying there, paralyzed. Not wanting to see his reaction, I left the room quickly and hurried down the hall. I had to separate myself from them.

When they came out of John's room, I led the way out to the parking lot. They had driven a long distance to stay such a short time. Carol helped her mother into the car and then walked back to where I stood waiting to say goodbye. As we talked, thinking that Carol, too, had been embarrassed by her mother's laughter, I whispered my concern to her.

But emotions were running high, and tempers flared at the slightest provocation. Instead of agreeing with me, Carol took offense. She had always been close to Jack, and she had thus been a constant in our lives, caring and supportive. Now, however, as the eldest of five children, she was keeping a protective arm around her aging parents. Angrily, she promptly yelled at me, "Don't you say anything about my mother!"

I pulled back from her, thinking, *Don't, Carol. I can't stand one more thing! I will collapse and never bounce back if anybody says one more angry thing to me!*

Suddenly, I felt and saw peripherally the wings of a guardian angel swoop down from behind me and envelop me protectively! Although Carol continued to scold me, the angel's wings covered my ears and I couldn't hear her. I could see her lips moving, but her words were unintelligible.

Simultaneously, I perceived that this guardian angel's wings, with feathers like those of a bird, were huge—perhaps seven or eight feet high—and that this angel was Dr. Hofmann! Stranger still, I learned later that Dr. Hofmann had not been at the hospital that Sunday afternoon!

Somehow comforted, I said nothing to Carol, and we waved goodbye as she drove off.

This incident foreshadowed another in which Dr. Hofmann's actual physical presence at St. Luke's was extremely crucial to me.

I have no explanation for what happened. Up until that time, the only angels that I had seen were in a picture in the bedroom that Sylvia and I shared as young girls. While I lay waiting for Sylvia to wake up in the morning, I often mused about the cherubs that appeared in the large gold-framed reproduction of a masterpiece that hung on the wall opposite my bed. Over the years, I had concluded that angels did not exist in real life, and that, in this instance, they were just a figment of the artist's imagination.

But following the incident in the parking lot, I decided that I would need to rethink the whole matter. I may not have believed in guardian angels, but I was quite sure about what I had seen and felt. Belief or no belief, I had definitely been saved by a guardian angel.

A Search in Vain

THE MERRIMENT

It is currently stated that hope goes with youth, and lends to youth its wings of a butterfly, but I fancy that hope is the last gift to man, and the only gift not given to youth. Youth is preeminently the period in which a man can be lyric, fanatical, poetic, but youth is the period in which a man can be hopeless. The end of every episode is the end of the world.

But the power of hoping through everything, the knowledge that the soul survives its adventures, this great inspiration comes to the middle-aged; God has kept this good wine until now. It is from the backs of the elderly gentlemen that the wings of the butterfly should burst. There is nothing that so much mystifies the young as the constant frivolity of the old. They have discovered their indestructibility. They are in their second and clearer childhood, and there is a meaning in the merriment of their eyes. They have seen the end of the End of the World.

-G. K. Chesterton

After giving us the prognosis following the second surgery, Dr. Hofmann suggested that we get a second opinion at the cancer center in Rockleigh. Pointing out that this center might be able to give us more updated information regarding the care and treatment of cancer, he referred us to Dr. Brooks, a neurosurgeon at University Hospital.

The following week, we left early one morning for Rockleigh. Only a few hours after John was admitted, however, we realized that this nationally renowned research facility did not deliver the personalized, loving care that St. Luke's had given us. With a maze of red and yellow lines in the corridors serving as our only means of direction, we were soon swallowed up in the vast compound.

Although we had an appointment with Dr. Brooks that morning, he did not come into the hospital that day. Nurses made several phone calls in an attempt to reach him, but their efforts were of no avail. Tired by 8 p.m., we left for the evening.

That night at our motel, Jack opened up to me and talked about John's predicament for the first time. He said he thought I blamed him for everything that had happened and that he therefore felt guilty.

I had known Jack since I was eight years old. We were classmates in school. I knew of his great love of sports and his fearlessness. I realized that he was reliving his youth through John when he had goaded him on to greater accomplishments. Thinking back to the time when John and his friends were trying out their homemade ski jump in the back yard, I knew that Jack would like to have been out on that hill himself.

I told Jack that I did not blame him. I knew that he meant well. To carry the blame for the death of one's child would be too heavy a burden for a loving parent to bear. Then, silently, I wondered why I had been forewarned about John's illness, yet could not stop it. Was it meant to happen? Did we all have a destiny?

Back at the hospital the next day, the nurses tried again in vain to locate Dr. Brooks. We asked if he had been called out of town. Were we waiting uselessly? By evening, at our insistence, nurses called his home and asked his wife of his whereabouts. She claimed to know nothing, so once more we left for the motel, tired and frustrated.

About 11 a.m. the next day, we finally met Dr. Brooks. Just as we arrived at John's room, he came out the door. After introducing ourselves, we mentioned that we'd been trying to locate him for two days.

"Oh, yes," he replied, "the nurses told me. Actually, I was over at the nursing home, visiting my mother."

Turning his attention back to his patient, he motioned toward John's door. "I've just examined your son. He's going to die. Does he know it?" he asked.

"Well, not exactly," I said. "The doctors told him after his second surgery that he'd never walk again. But that's as far as it's gone."

Hardly listening, Dr. Brooks said adamantly, "Well, I'm going back in there and tell him right now."

"Oh, no, doctor, don't do that," I pleaded. "He's in good shape psychologically, and I wouldn't want to spoil that." After John's surgery for the second tumor, in a joint effort with the staff at St. Luke's, we had supplied him with plenty of love and laughter to boost his spirits, and he was thriving on it. To destroy that now would destroy all of us.

When I saw that Dr. Brooks was not convinced, I continued, "How many times do we have to be told that John is going to die, and how many times does he have to be told? We all know it already. We've been told several times, and he has, too—indirectly. I don't think we should destroy hope. Hope keeps us going."

"No," the doctor insisted, moving toward the door. "I'm going in there and tell him."

I raised my voice in anger. "Dr. Brooks, I'm ordering you not to. He is our son, and we don't want him upset any more! We just can't take it! We want to go home. Just let us out of here."

Dr. Brooks turned back toward us. "All right," he said. With an angry look in his eyes, he added, "I'll arrange for your discharge." He then turned and strode away from us down the corridor.

Jack and I walked to the end of the hall, where we collapsed into two leather chairs near the window. I could not talk now. Putting my hand on my chest as I gasped for breath, I tried to signal to Jack that I needed an aspirin. He left and came back with a nurse, who was empty-handed.

"What is the problem, Mrs. Redmond?" the nurse asked.

I couldn't answer. Breathing heavily, I motioned to Jack and mouthed the word "aspirin."

"We can't give you aspirin, Mrs. Redmond," the nurse said.

I raised my eyebrows questioningly. Aspirin was an over-the-counter medicine.

"You might be allergic to it," she continued.

I shook my head to tell her that I wasn't. I often took aspirin now to quiet my nerves.

But she just stood there, silent.

Through Jack, I managed to convey to the nurse that any substitute would do. I had to have something.

"I can give you Tylenol," she replied finally.

Still gasping, I nodded.

Shortly, she came back with the pill and a glass of water. But she left the moment I swallowed it. For another half-hour we sat alone, until I felt able to walk back to John's room. The doctor had discharged him, so we left for home immediately. All three of us were considerably relieved to be out of there.

***

The task of caring for John at home became burdensome, and a series of admissions and discharges at St. Luke's followed. Our level of emotional involvement with our son was so intense that it sapped our energy to care for him physically. Although Jack worked full-time, he set the alarm every night to get up and turn John every two hours. I handled his daytime care, along with attending to the needs of the family. A visiting nurse stopped in twice a week to check on John.

Dr. Hofmann told us that John would eventually have to go to a nursing home, since St. Luke's was an acute-care facility. Knowing that this would be a blow to John, we sidestepped the issue, hoping that time would obviate the need to deal with it. John had formed a close bond with the caregivers at St. Luke's during his long-term illness. His problems had become their problems, and he thrived on their attention and concern. We feared that a nursing home might be too depressing for such a young person.

Unfortunately, hospice care was not an option at that time. The first hospice in the United States was established in 1974,[9] one year after John died.

---

[9] Under the direction of the Hospice Education Committee, of which the author was a member, the groundwork was laid to establish a hospice in Dickinson in 1978.

All Downhill

In March of 1973, while John was in St. Luke's Hospital, Jack jumped out of bed in the middle of the night and headed for the bathroom. When I heard him vomiting, I assumed that he was coming down with the flu, which was almost of epidemic proportions in our area. But when he got back into bed and I heard him struggling for breath, I sensed that something else might be wrong.

Not wanting to alarm him or to waken the children, I quietly got up and called the emergency room of Cobourg Hospital. The attendant there told me to bring Jack right down. Although I have no recollection of it, I must have driven him to the hospital.

Jack had had a heart attack, and during the three weeks he was recovering, I visited both my husband and my son in two hospitals twenty miles apart. On some days, I managed to see only one of them. Following his release, Jack recuperated another six weeks at home.

When I called Rob to tell him about his father's heart attack, he came home immediately. He was in his junior year at the University of Southern Illinois. A few days later, he surprised us by offering to stay home and manage the business while Jack was recuperating.

Rob had worked with his father intermittently throughout high school and his first two years of college. He felt confident that he could do the job with the help of Carl, our employee. Although we were concerned about his missing the spring semester, Rob assured us that he needed some time off anyway. He said he was sick of school. His generosity eased our burden.

Earl, Rob's paternal grandfather, was a man of modest means who kept a watchful eye on his children. Having worked for the Federal Land Bank, he knew the value of paying cash, with no interest payments. Over the years, he generously gave loans to his children at four percent when they were needed, and he imposed no time restrictions on repayment. When he heard of Rob's offer to manage our business temporarily, he was overjoyed, exclaiming, "He'll be rewarded in heaven for this unselfish act!"

When we told Rob about his grandfather's comment, he was embarrassed. Laughing, he replied, "Grandpa must think they keep track of good deeds in heaven and give you brownie points!" To Rob, this was an absurdity.

But years later, I read a book by Betty J. Eadie in which she related her near-death experience. She said that when she met Jesus, a film of her life unreeled before her, and she learned that every kind or unkind act she had performed in her life had caused a pronounced effect on others. Thus, she was required to judge the impact of her behavior—for good or ill—on those around her.[10]

After Jack returned to work, his doctor told me privately that although he had not restricted him in his lifestyle or diet, he might have a second, fatal heart attack in four years. Unable to cope with more than one day at a time, I rejected his prognosis. I did not have the strength to face the loss of two loved ones simultaneously. In order to spare our children, I did not tell them, hoping that the doctor would be mistaken.

***

In June 1973, John, now totally bedridden, lost weight and became weaker. Suffering from nausea, he was unable to retain food. When the staff insisted that he eat his favorite ham sandwiches for lunch in order to maintain his strength, the outcome was always the same. After he ate, he vomited. It seemed senseless to me to keep repeating this procedure. But the nurses explained that even though John threw up most of the food, he

---

10 Betty J. Eadie, *Embraced by the Light*, Placerville, California: Gold Leaf Press, 1992.

retained enough to sustain him. They measured the amount that he lost in order to determine what he had gained.

As I watched daily, I began to reminisce about earlier days, when Dr. O'Bryan, a white-haired man in his sixties, was our family physician. He kept his patients waiting an hour or two past their appointment time, but they were tolerant of his lateness. They thought of him as a friend, so they valued the time he took to visit with them when they did get to see him.

As I sat in his office one day bouncing John on my lap, I made a wish that haunted me years later. Dr. O'Bryan asked me if the rash I'd had for six months had ever cleared up. I had endured internal itching, for which there seemed to be no help, even after securing six different opinions from six different doctors.

I told Dr. O'Bryan that a gynecologist had finally solved the problem in one office visit. He'd diagnosed it as an allergy to penicillin and prescribed a cream that worked right away. Penicillin was the new wonder drug on the market, and doctors, not realizing its potency, used it as a cure-all. Dr. O'Bryan had given me several shots of penicillin for my recurring sore throats.

"Doctors make me sick," I grumbled to Dr. O'Bryan, thinking that even if two of the six doctors had agreed, I would have recovered sooner. "You couldn't find two doctors to agree on ANYTHING! I wish they'd make up their minds!"

For a moment, Dr. O'Bryan just gazed out the window. Then he turned toward me and nodded in agreement. "That's right, Barbara, doctors do disagree," he said good-naturedly. After a pause, he added, "When two doctors agree—you're dead!" We laughed heartily at this new twist he put upon it.

Years later, I finally got my wish. That night up on the fourth floor of St. Luke's, I finally heard two doctors agree—on the death of my son—John, that child I'd bounced on my lap while we were laughing that day in Dr. O'Bryan's office!

Then, too, I remembered another time when the good doctor helped me through a bout with the children's old-fashioned measles. When I was trying to cope with their constant nausea, he had advised, "Stop the solid food! Just give them liquids!" It had worked! Now it made me wonder. Would that approach be effective in this case?

One day, when we were alone, I asked John how he felt about eating. "I don't want to eat," he said, "but the nurses make me. They say I have to eat to keep up my strength!" When I told him about the advice Dr. O'Bryan had given me years earlier, he said that he would like to try it. When I apprised Dr. Hofmann of the situation later that day, he agreed to restrict John's diet to liquids only.

Immediately, nurses and aides gave me hostile looks to express their disapproval of the order. One of John's most loyal caregivers, fiery Marcia, acted out her displeasure. Coming up from behind, she passed me in the hall with her head held erect and chin up. Stretching her five-foot-frame to a tall, rigid position, she took exaggerated strides, as if she were Charles de Gaulle marching down the Champs-Elysées. Apparently I was invading their territory.

Her actions made me wish that I could take John home, where I could care for him as I pleased. Unfortunately, this was not possible.

With the temperature nearing 100 degrees, I ran to the parking lot. It was suffocating inside the car, but I didn't wait for the air conditioning to take effect. I was hardly able to touch the scorching steering wheel, but I headed for the Convenient Food Mart, where I bought containers of yogurt and several small cans of grapefruit and orange juice. Then I hurried back to the hospital. I felt better now. My hands were no longer tied. Finally, I could do something!

At dinnertime, John drank the juice through a straw, and I gave him sips of it several times throughout the evening. Within a few days, the vomiting stopped, and he was able to retain both the juice and the yogurt. By the end of the week, I sighed. We had prevailed through one more crisis.

***

On the Fourth of July, John celebrated his sixteenth birthday in the hospital. While I was at lunch, my friend Nancy and her daughter, Sue, made a surprise visit. They trimmed John's room with red, white, and blue streamers and brought him a large birthday cake decorated with the Stars and Stripes.

Although John could not eat the cake, nurses, aides, and orderlies joined him in his room that evening to celebrate. Staff members whom we had never seen before showed up to banter with John while they ate the cake. John, Jack, and I enjoyed the festivities. We were sorely in need of some merriment.

***

A few weeks later, because of the unrelenting temperatures and high humidity, Dr. Hofmann moved John to an air-conditioned room on the rehabilitation floor in the new wing of the hospital. Bedridden patients such as John who lay on rubber sheets for prolonged periods of time suffered the most discomfort from the heat.

Shortly thereafter, John began to have violent headaches. Nurses applied cold compresses to his forehead, but when they did not afford relief, Dr. Hofmann told us that nothing further could be done to alleviate the pain. Over time, the doctor explained, as the tumor in John's spinal cord slowly moved up to his brain, the headaches would continue to get worse. In addition, he would eventually lose his eyesight.

John's pain was so intense that I periodically had to leave the room. I could not bear the sound of his moaning. After he lost his eyesight, he did not want to be alone, so we worked out shifts. I stayed with him from 9 a.m. to 6 p.m., alternating between the hall and his room. Jack kept him company during the evening until Lynn arrived at 10 to assume the night vigil. She dozed in a chair in John's room until the morning, when hospital staff members came in to feed and bathe him.

***

During the long stretch of John's illness, I hired a cleaning woman, Betty, to come in biweekly to help me with the housework. Her husband was a minister in the Jehovah's Witnesses church. They had three children to support, and she worked to supplement her husband's small salary.

As I worked alongside Betty, we visited and shared our problems. Each time she came to clean, she would ask about John. When I told her that the doctors could provide no relief for his excruciating headaches, she said, "You ought to try the grape diet."

"The grape diet!" I exclaimed. "What's that?"

"It's a diet that some of our church members use to cure cancer," she answered.

"Cure cancer?" I repeated, disbelieving. There was no cure for cancer. Didn't Betty know that?

However, she insisted that she had tried the diet herself a few years before, when she had a malignant lump in her breast. The lump had disappeared, and since then she'd had no problems. She knew of others in her church who had used the diet successfully. When she offered to borrow the book from a friend so that I could read it, I agreed, but I remained skeptical.

The small hardcover book, *The Grape Cure,*[11] had been published in 1928, and it showed the effects of extensive use. In it, author Johanna

---

11 Only in 1995, when I began an arduous search for this out-of-print book to cite it properly in this text did I learn that a revised edition is still in print: Johanna Brandt, N.D., *How to Conquer Cancer Naturally (The Grape Cure),* Joshua Tree, California: Tree of Life Publications, 1989, 1996. (See Appendix.)

Brandt, a doctor of naturopathy, revealed that she had successfully used the cure on herself after a nine-year bout with stomach cancer. Leaving her husband and young children behind, she eagerly began a journey on the Fourth of July, 1927, from her home in South Africa to share her discovery with the medical profession in the United States.

She wrote, "America was a free country politically, and an independent, powerful, progressive, rich and enlightened nation. But it was not free from disease. I had no doubt whatsoever that this free nation would accept my message, and, accepting it, be blessed with a new emancipation—a wonderful deliverance from disease and premature death."

An astrologer who attended a lecture given by Dr. Brandt in Cape Town advised her to abandon her trip because planetary influences were against the enterprise. Dr. Brandt pressed on, however, feeling that she would overcome any negative influences by the grace of God. Indeed, she believed that her discovery of the grape diet was "the direct result of Divine Illumination."

While staying with a friend in New York, she addressed the medical community, but she was devastated to find that "the Medical Practice Act of the State of New York was tyrannical in the extreme." Only two individuals who attended her lecture encouraged her to continue. One was a surgeon of exceptionally high standing, and the other was a natural health pioneer, Bernarr Macfadden, who later published an article by Dr. Brandt in his famous magazine *Physical Culture.*

After receiving positive feedback on her article, Dr. Brandt established a test clinic, where she used her mono-diet of organic grapes on volunteer cancer patients at no charge. Although she demonstrated a high survival rate, she was extremely disappointed that she did not receive support from American doctors. Eventually she returned to her home in South Africa, where she opened a clinic and earned many testimonials following favorable outcomes.

Still uncertain, I returned the book to Betty. A few days later, my brother Don called from California to inquire about John. I filled him in on the sad turn of events but, afraid that he might ridicule me, I did not mention the grape diet. My older brother had a compassionate heart, but he was also a big tease.

Strangely, he proceeded to ask me if I had ever heard of it. When I told him that I had just finished reading a book about it, he said that a friend had recently told him that he'd had great success with it. His doctor couldn't believe it when X-rays taken following the grape diet showed no signs of the malignant tumor.

"I just thought I'd call and tell you about it," Don said. "It might be worth your while to try it." Pausing, he added, "Of course, it's *your* decision."

For a few more days, I watched John's suffering. When I could stand it no longer, I borrowed the book from Betty once more and asked Jack to read it. Jack was noncommittal, however. He held little hope for John's recovery.

But I could not let go. One day, a new nurse on the floor came over to me as I was sitting at the end of the hall near John's room. Putting her hand on my shoulder, she said sympathetically, "It must be very hard on you."

I told her that it was, adding that I was experiencing a difficult inner struggle that I did not understand. "All outward signs point to the fact that John is going to die," I said, "and those around me do not understand why I won't believe that. It's common knowledge that there is no cure for cancer. Yet a voice within me contradicts this and tells me he is going to live. It's very hard to contend with. I feel torn by it."

Then I thought about how hard it might be to convince John that any variation from the conventional medicine he'd seen practiced on *Medical Center* would help him. In these times, parents had little credibility. I feared that he might prefer the medical staff's word to his mother's.

Finally, I took a deep breath and plunged in. Squatting beside John's bed to make eye contact with him, I told him about the book on the grape diet and the wonderful results from the research on it. Next, I told him that if he decided to try it, it might serve a twofold purpose. First, it would be nourishment for him, since he could not retain solid food. Second, if it did flush the toxins from his system, as the book claimed it would, it might alleviate his suffering from the headaches.

To my surprise, John agreed to try it. I sighed, relieved, and left the room quickly, before I could say anything that might spoil it. I felt more spirited now, more hopeful.

The next day, I handed the book to Dr. Hofmann and asked him to read it, suggesting that he might have time to do so in the quiet early morning hours. Nurses had told me that he stayed at the hospital all night. He was an extremely busy man, one who was constantly being paged over the loudspeaker.

A few days later, Dr. Hofmann handed the book back to me without comment. When I asked him what he thought about the diet, he raised his eyebrows, gave me a half-smile, and shrugged his shoulders.

Realizing that he might be concerned about his reputation, I said, "Well, after all, Dr. Hofmann, there is nothing to lose. You've given him only four weeks to live. It certainly can't hurt him. It's not as if we would be giving him strong drugs. It's just grapes and grape juice."

Quietly, he nodded in agreement. "I know, but you can't administer the diet with no medication. It would be inhumane to take his pain medication away from him."

"Oh, I know," I agreed. "We couldn't do that to him." I knew that the instructions pertaining to the diet stated that it should not be accompanied by medication of any kind. But I also knew that we were starting the program in a very late stage of John's illness.

"My friend says it really works, Dr. Hofmann," I insisted.

"Yeah? Well, you try telling the Surgeon General that," he replied. "You know, I'm leaving soon. I'm going to Austria for six weeks. I won't be here."

"I can do it," I pleaded. "All I need is permission to feed him." Hesitating, I added, "I know the nurses won't agree with it."

"Never mind," he said. "I'll handle that." Then he ventured, "You'll have to have access to a refrigerator that isn't often used to store the grapes.

Otherwise, you'll lose them. I'll have to move you off the rehab floor. You'll lose your air-conditioned room."

"That's all right. We'll manage," I replied eagerly.

Hours later, Dr. Hofmann issued an order for aides to move John to the fourth floor. He put a notation on John's chart that, effective immediately, I was the only one allowed to feed him.

The next day, I met with Bill Snyder, the hospital's social worker, who helped me solve daily problems. A long-term patient's survival on the hospital floor was difficult. With fewer registered nurses working on the floor, and eight-hour shift changes, misunderstandings often erupted between the patient, the family, and/or the licensed practical nurses and other staff members.

As we talked, Mr. Snyder picked up the grape diet book from his desk. "I perused your book," he said casually. I was surprised. Thinking that Dr. Hofmann had betrayed my confidence, I was also angry. I feared the social worker's opposition. But there was none, and later I realized that Dr. Hofmann had told Mr. Snyder about our new procedure so that he could protect me if problems arose during the doctor's absence.

As we were leaving the hospital that night, Jack and I met Dr. Hofmann in the hallway. Jack told the doctor that putting John on the grape diet made no sense to him. Jack had been raised by conventional methods of medicine, and he continued to believe in them exclusively.

Conversely, a mother who believed in finding her own remedies for ailments had raised me. Although it was uncommon to take vitamins when I was growing up, she took them and gave them to Sylvia and me, along with cod-liver oil.

My mother based her decisions on recommendations made by Dr. William Brady in his syndicated newspaper column. Dr. Brady, who was ahead of his time in believing that vitamins and calcium could be a source of healing and good health, educated his readers on how and when to use them. Although his credentials were never published in his column, he had his followers, and my mother was one of them.

She also believed in spiritual healing. When Sylvia and I were in grade school, she hung scapular medals around our necks to ward off scarlet fever. We wore them unwillingly, believing them to be the product of our mother's superstitious nature. We were thankful, though, that we could wear them under our sweaters. Our schoolmates would have ridiculed us if they had been able to see them.

Even though my parents square-danced in the same set with Dr. Foster and his wife almost every week, and Dr. Foster had delivered both Sylvia and me at home, my healthy mother shied away from doctors and hospitals. She told us that her mother had feared doctors and hospitals. At that time, doctors unknowingly were still spreading germs with their hands.

That night at the hospital, when Jack expressed concern to Dr. Hofmann about my using the grape diet, I was gratified by the doctor's response. "Oh, let her do it," he urged Jack. "She's just grasping at straws."

That was a crucial moment. It tore at my heart to see my child in such pain while I stood by, unable to help him. Dr. Hofmann must have understood my *need* to try another approach. By this kind act, he may have preserved my sanity.

The next day, he left for Austria.

***

A few weeks later, Don called again to see how things were going. When I told him that we had started John on the grape diet, both of us expressed astonishment at the perfect timing of his first call. We marveled at how this could happen with 3,000 miles between us. We had not talked with each other in the past few months, then suddenly we were both thinking along the same lines about a little-known topic! Finally, we shrugged if off as "another unexplainable coincidence."

Nevertheless, after talking with Don, I felt more confident that I had chosen the right path.

Letting Go

One day, Father Cyril stopped me in the hall and told me that I should talk with John. "He wants to die," he said bluntly. Shaken, I questioned him further about how he knew this. All he would say was, "We had a talk yesterday, and he told me." Father Cyril had given me a lecture previously about letting John die. "Everyone has a right to die!" he insisted. But Father Cyril was talking to the wrong person. I would have thrown myself in front of a truck, if necessary, to save my child from danger.

Nevertheless, a day or two later, I sat by John's bedside, waiting to hear what was on his mind. Following his first surgery, I had never understood why he was so complacent about his illness. Aware of the mind/body connection, I thought that if he refused to accept his condition, it would boost his immune system.

One day, I confronted him about it. "Why aren't you angry about what's happened to you, John?" I asked.

Shrugging his shoulders, he reasoned, "Well, there's nothing I can do about it, Mom, so I might as well accept it."

"But you can't die, John, because I couldn't stand it!" I argued. I knew that the thought of losing a child was my Achilles' heel.

Now, as I sat with John and listened, he complained for the first time. He began by telling me that neither the nurses nor the aides would turn him in bed when he asked them to do so. Sometimes he had to wait a half-hour before they arrived. Thirty minutes can be a long time to wait when one is in an uncomfortable position.

Finally, he said simply, "I want to die." I looked at his thin frame as he lay there, helpless. I reached for his hand and held it. I had not realized that he was so frustrated, and I asked myself, *What kind of life was this to lie in bed helplessly and have to beg someone to turn you?* And from the depths of my heart, I replied quietly, "I don't blame you, honey. I understand. If I were in your position, I wouldn't want to live either."

Only later did I realize that in order to die, John would have to have my blessing. I had to let go.

The Long, Hot Summer

In the older part of the hospital, the private room at the end of the hall had only one small window. To help offset the sweltering temperatures outside, I bought a twenty-inch table fan in downtown Dickinson. We stored the grapes, grape juice, and spring water in a refrigerator in a tiny room across the hall.

Although Marcia had a sincere love for John, she strongly opposed my using the grape diet, so I could not trust her. She had considerable influence over John, and in those times, I, as a parent, had little or no credibility and authority. Therefore, at my request, Dr. Hofmann restricted visitors to family and family friends only. We were trying an unconventional treatment in a traditional setting, and I hoped to avoid opposition.

Since the grape cure required the patient to fast for the first two days on pure, cold water, I bought spring water for John to drink. It was not yet customary to buy bottled water for drinking. The public had only recently been informed about impurities in tap water. I found the spring water so refreshing in the hot temperatures that John and I drank it together.

After two days on water, in order to flush toxins from the body, the patient was required to drink grape juice or to eat grapes at three-hour intervals, twelve hours a day, for six to eight weeks, depending on the stage of the illness. Since John's illness was in an advanced stage, I thought that he needed to stay on the diet for eight weeks. The book warned that even though the patient might beg for food toward the end of the diet, studies had proven that it was better to hold off until the designated time period had expired.

I bought the grapes and grape juice at a nearby supermarket, and from 9 a.m. to 9 p.m. I fed John, taking breaks when he slept and when the nurses were bathing him and changing his bedding.

Although the doctor had told me that John's headaches would get worse instead of better, the pain stopped within three days. I was able to stay in the room with him, passing the time reading or working on a crewel picture that I had never finished.

Until this time, John had been paralyzed from about two inches above the waist down. Just as we started the grape diet, he lost the use of his arms. However, during the second week of the diet, he was able to use them again. It had been impossible for him to sleep on his back for two and a half years—since his first tumor surgery—but after another week on the diet, he could lie on his back and sleep peacefully.

Throughout this period, Jack's family remained faithful, coming down every weekend from three directions—Stonehill, Lookout Point, and Middletown. Close friends shied away, however, fearful of saying the wrong thing. Total strangers often approached me in the grocery and drugstore in Cobourg to tell me that their prayer group was praying for us. This was comforting news. I had not been aware that John's present circumstances were well known in our hometown.

When Dr. Hofmann returned from Austria at the end of six weeks, John was resting comfortably, free from pain and nausea. After examining him, the doctor stood by the door of his room, talking with me. Beaming across the room at his patient, he said excitedly, "He's better! His condition has much improved!" Even though John was still blind, he turned toward the door and beamed right back at Dr. Hofmann. That old rapport between them continued.

A few days later, John surprised me. Although I had informed him at the outset about the length of time he would have to remain on the diet, he asked me if he could have some solid food. I recalled reading the book,

Fasting Can Save Your Life.[12] It reported that, in 1963, two plane crash victims had survived for seven weeks in bitterly cold weather with little or no food. In the last six of those weeks, they had nothing but water. Following their rescue, physicians had noted that they were in "remarkably good" condition. Based on this account, I was confident that fasting would not hurt John.

But his request for food now gave me pause. I thought about how much we had invested in his diet. For twelve hours daily throughout the last six weeks, I had sat with him, brought him spring water and grapes and grape juice, and fed him. Lynn had sat up with him at night, and Rob and Jack had relieved intermittently. What if two more weeks would make all the difference between success and failure? If the headaches and nausea returned, did any of us have the strength to cope with them? Couldn't we remain in this pain-free, peaceful cocoon forever?

I begged John to stay on the grapes and grape juice just two more weeks. Because he did not argue, I believed that he had accepted my advice. But I should have known that when a sixteen-year-old boy is hungry, he will beg, borrow, or steal to get food. If John had been able to walk, he would have grabbed a leftover from the refrigerator when I was out of the room—or, staring me down boldly, he would have eaten the food right in front of me.

Since this was not possible, he had only one alternative. At night, after I had left the hospital, he begged his sister for food. It tore at Lynn's heart to have to refuse him. The day she came home from the hospital and talked to me about it, I told her that I believed the most beneficial thing we could do was hold John off, as the book recommended. She did not argue with me.

---

12 Herbert M. Shelton, *Fasting Can Save Your Life*, Chicago: Natural Hygiene Press, 1964.

Although John and I had only the one conversation about stopping the diet, one night shortly thereafter, while Jack and Lynn were there, the nurses brought him a plate of spaghetti. When Jack came home, he told me that John had eaten. He insisted that this one meal couldn't hurt, adding that it was cruel to refuse a dying child food.

Although I said nothing, I was dismayed that the nurses had fed John. Who made the decision to take him off the diet? No one had informed me that the doctor had altered his orders. Had he really changed his mind? Sadly, I never got a chance to look into the matter.

The next morning, like an angry bear trying to protect her cub from danger, I stood by John's bed with my hands on my hips and glared down at him. "Well, John," I said, "I hear you had a plate of spaghetti last night! You know you shouldn't eat yet. You might get sick again!"

With eyes closed, John replied defiantly, "I'll eat anytime I want to." This did not sound like John! Had someone coached him?

It was as if a red flag had been waved in front of me. I charged blindly. Reaching down, I slapped his face—the only part of his body outside the covers. I felt betrayed. Then I marched out of the room and went home.

That night, Jack brought me a message from the hospital. From that time on, I could not be alone with John. I would have to be accompanied by another adult each time I visited, and that visit could last only one hour. Hospital security guards would be placed outside the door of John's room to enforce the order. In addition, I was told to call and make an appointment with Dr. Hirsch, a psychiatrist who had been called in on the case.

PARIAH

Dr. Hirsch startled me. His secretary had instructed me to meet him in an open area of the hospital. But no sooner had I introduced myself to the doctor, a dark-haired man in his fifties who stood more than six feet tall, than he started yelling at me. What did I think I was doing—slapping my invalid son? Why was I putting him on a grape diet? Didn't I understand that there was no cure for malignant cancer?

Embarrassed, I glanced behind me. Patients and visitors were coming and going near the elevator. I hadn't expected to meet the doctor in such a public space. In hushed tones, I asked, "Dr. Hirsch, isn't there some other place we can discuss this?"

"No," he replied in a loud voice. "We'll discuss it right here!"

He continued to berate me until Dr. Mitchell, the plastic surgeon who had performed surgery on John's bedsore, suddenly appeared on the scene. Standing beside me, he glowered at Dr. Hirsch for a moment, then looked at me and said, "Mrs. Redmond, is there anything that I can do for you?"

Shocked and humiliated, when I realized that he had overheard Dr. Hirsch's accusations, I thanked him kindly but declined his invitation to help. I had great respect for this man, and I didn't want him to think ill of me. As he turned to leave, he gave Dr. Hirsch a look as if to say, Cool it, man. What are you doing to this woman who has been looking after her son every day for more than two years? Are you crazy?

Frantically looking around, I spotted an empty office through a transparent glass wall. "Dr. Hirsch," I said, "why can't we discuss this matter in there?"

Having been admonished by a colleague, Dr. Hirsch led the way into the office. Scanning the room, he positioned himself with his back against some bookshelves, like an armed policeman confronting a dangerous criminal. I stood, facing him. He looked out through the glass wall to see if he was visible to passers-by. Then he launched into another tirade. Never questioning me as to what had happened, he repeatedly threatened to have me committed to a mental institution.

Instead of accusing me this way, I thought that he ought to be telling me that he would support me in any way he could. Finally, I interrupted him. "Dr. Hirsch, you haven't even heard my side of the story. You don't know what I've been through for the last two and a half years trying to save John. I've been fighting the odds daily. Don't you understand? I'm his mother! Who called you in anyway?"

Not waiting for an answer, I continued, "Well, I didn't, so don't send me any bills. I'm not paying them because you're not helping me!" Turning on my heel defiantly, I walked out. Our meeting had lasted less than ten minutes.

That evening, not knowing what might transpire, I called my brother Joe and told him about the confrontation. Joe had recently taken early retirement from a full professorship at the State University of Riverside, and he was now secretary of a professional licensing board for the State Education Department.

When Joe and his wife, Peg, had visited us at the hospital just a few weeks before, I had explained the grape diet and told him about Don's friend in California who had tried it with great results. Although Joe was noncommittal, he agreed that, under the circumstances, it certainly couldn't hurt John.

Joe called Dr. Hofmann the next day. After introducing himself as my brother, he said, "Now, you guys aren't going to put her in any mental institution because she's not crazy! She told me about the grape diet when I was down there a couple of weeks ago. She's just as sane as you and I are, so tell that psychiatrist to lay off! Frankly, I don't know how she keeps going under the circumstances!"

Joe phoned me that night to tell me not to worry. He had taken care of the matter.

Broken-hearted and feeling defeated, I went upstairs to Rob's empty bedroom. I needed solitude. Suffering from total exhaustion, I slept for an entire week, getting up only to shower and to eat leftovers from the dinner that Lynn had fixed the night before.

Fortunately Lynn liked to cook, and she excelled at it. During those six weeks of twelve-hour days that I had spent at the hospital, she had fixed meals morning and night for Jack and Christopher. Following her graduation from high school in June, she had started working behind the lunch counter at a neighborhood drugstore. After work each day, she went to the hospital at 10 p.m. to relieve Jack and to keep the night vigil. Distraught about her brother's predicament, she had him on her mind constantly.

A Time to Reflect

While I was home that week, I called Sister Sheila Rourke to tell her about my dilemma. A nun from the Sisters of St. Joseph, she now worked in Rockleigh. We had maintained a close friendship ever since she'd taught my children in sixth grade at St. Patrick's School in Cobourg.

T*he Documents of Vatican II*, which had been published in 1966, stated that the laity would need to play a greater role in the church. At the time, Sheila, much like Maria von Trapp in *The Sound of Music*, was having misgivings about her usefulness in the confines of the convent. Therefore, as soon as the church condoned her wearing street clothes, she shed her black habit in the belief that it separated her from the layperson, whom she desperately wanted to help.

We were living in chaotic times of change in the church. Authorities encouraged both laity and clergy to shed their masks and reveal their true identities. For the first time in the church's history, clergymen became involved in political and civil-rights issues. With the help of the laity, they battered away at long-held traditions, which divided church members. Irreverence reigned, resulting in untold suffering and misery.

In our telephone conversation, I told Sheila that only she could comprehend my predicament. With little confidence now, I felt deceived and hurt. Though I yearned to see John again, I was considering removing myself from the situation.

When Sheila arrived in Cobourg at the end of the week, she told me about Father Martin Braun at Mount Saviour Monastery. Describing him as a "wonderful, understanding, compassionate man who had been a urologist before becoming a scholastic," she asked me if I would meet with him if she could arrange it. She believed that he could grasp the complexity of my situation, which involved both medicine and spirituality.

Primarily, she explained, Father Braun functioned as a counselor for troubled priests in the diocese. Women were not allowed to enter the monastery, but perhaps he would make an exception in my case.

When I agreed to go, Sheila called him, and they made an appointment for us to meet the next day.

The monastery, which was located back in the woods on a hillside, was less than ten miles from my home. I had driven past the white arrow-shaped sign leading to Mount Saviour whenever I had taken the shortcut to the hospital, but I had hardly noticed it.

As I stepped out of the car that day, I paused to absorb the breathtaking beauty of the natural surroundings. There, even the air was refreshing, and I inhaled deep breaths of it. As I moved forward hesitantly through the entranceway, I took in the gilt-framed oils on the walls, which had been signed by one of the brothers.

In the sunlit dining room, I noticed the simple plank floors as I passed a long mission-type table surrounded by high-backed wooden chairs. Looking out through a sun-streaked window, I saw sheep grazing in green pastures. It was like a scene from an artist's canvas. Huge aqua glass bottles filled with purple and gold wildflowers occupied the space in two corners of the room.

To the left, all four walls of the huge library were covered with floor-to-ceiling bookshelves overflowing with books and pamphlets. Off to the right, through an open door, I saw a small chapel.

Father Braun greeted me and took me back to his office. His calm manner was comforting, and after we had talked a while, I felt more centered. Here was a man close to nature and God's goodness, a man who assured me that I was not crazy to have tried the grape diet on my son. Hadn't early man survived solely on fruit and berries? He asked me if he could read the book on the grape diet.

He said that it was of the utmost importance for me to go back to the hospital to be with my son. Wisely reminding me that I could not care for John at home, he advised me to defer to the doctors' treatment.

Throughout our conversation, I remarked several times how serene it was at the monastery. Father Braun noted that Vietnam veterans had often stayed there for as long as a year in order to collect their thoughts and to meditate on the future.

As I stepped back outside that morning, the heat of the late August sun warmed my body. The early morning dew glistened on the rolling green pastures, and the sight of glorious magenta, burgundy, and gold mums lining a stone wall lifted my spirits as I walked along the pathway to the car.

Living in a period when it was fashionable to replace real flowers and plants in homes and offices with artificial ones that required no water, I realized that nature was a life-giving source of energy. Like a released prisoner of war too long consumed by my need for self-preservation, I reveled in the joy of simple pleasures. Just *being* at the monastery had revitalized me.

Later that week, Jack brought me a message from Dr. Hofmann. He said that I should come back to the hospital. John wanted to see me, and there wasn't much time left.

***

Sheila and I visited John every afternoon, passing the two uniformed guards in light gray trousers and gray short-sleeved shirts who sat dutifully in the hall outside the door. When Sheila had to return to Rockleigh occasionally, I asked friends or neighbors to accompany me to the hospital. If they declined because they were busy, I was forced to tell them that it was urgent because I could not go alone. Not understanding, they asked, "Why not? Aren't you his mother?" I made a few excuses, but I did not elaborate. It was such a long story, and too painful to discuss. Fortunately, they complied without further questions.

Jack went to the hospital in the evening after work, but visits from Lynn, who was now a freshman at Cobourg Community College, were infrequent. In addition to her studies, she was working part-time at the drugstore. We lived one day at a time, and each day John became weaker.

Eventually, Dr. Hofmann moved John to a pediatric ward, where a new staff took over his care. Sheila and I visited him in the afternoon, and I learned through the hospital network that Marcia saw him every day after she got off work. Early on, for pain management, shots of Demerol administered every three hours kept him comfortable. But towards the end, after two hours, he would start asking if it was time for another injection.

Five weeks passed. John then developed pneumonia.

The Final Call

When the phone rang at nine o'clock that September morning, I was alone. The caller, a hospital staff member, told me that John had died in his sleep during the night.

Quietly, I hung up the phone and stared out the kitchen window. Trying to absorb the shock, I stood numb and lifeless, gazing at the quarter-acre of land behind our house. Suddenly, hundreds—or was it thousands—of starlings swooped down and landed on our lawn. They seemed to cover every blade of grass. Not wanting to frighten them away, I held my breath and did not move. I watched them feed there for several moments.

The sight was hard to believe, but the timing was perfect. Years before, I had seen a similar scene during Alfred Hitchcock's movie *The Birds*. But that was fiction. This time, it was real. I saw it with my own eyes.

After a few moments, I telephoned Jack. Within an hour, we met with Sister Ignatius at the hospital. As we walked down the corridor together, she asked me if I would like to see John, pointing out that he was in a room nearby. When she noticed the startled look on my face, she explained, "I just thought you'd like to see the beautiful smile on his face. He looks so peaceful."

I declined, saying that I didn't believe I could handle it. What I didn't say was that I feared that if I looked at him, I might break down and never recover.

***

Two days later, during calling hours at the funeral home, several of St. Luke's caregivers, including Marcia, told me that as John lay paralyzed in bed, he counseled them on their personal problems. When I indicated that I did not understand—John was just a young boy—they countered with, "Quite the contrary." They insisted that he was wise beyond his years and that he had given them workable solutions to their concerns.

Two young girls related how upset Sara Holton had been all through John's illness. Although I was unaware of it, Sara and some of her seventh-grade classmates had visited John several times at the hospital. Her father, a millionaire, was the chief executive officer of a worldwide corporation headquartered in Cobourg. According to the girls, Sara had had a crush on John ever since she'd met him in middle school.

I knew none of this, but I did recall that John had attended a pizza party at Sara's house before he became ill. When he told me matter-of-factly that Sara had handed him an invitation at school, I did not want to spoil an innocent relationship, so I did not mention her father's great wealth or position in the community. Apparently, John never caught on.

The day after the party, I had asked, "What did you think of their house, John?" The Holtons' home was filled with beautiful art objects from around the world. In addition, everyone in the community had a deep respect for the family's compassion and philanthropic efforts.

Shrugging, John had replied nonchalantly, "Oh, it was OK."

"How was the party?"

"Oh, great! We had a good time!" Like any twelve-year-old boy, John enthused about the pizza and fun while remaining oblivious to the interior décor of a millionaire's home.

The funeral home was crowded for two afternoons and two evenings. We kept going on the hugs and love poured out to us from family, friends, and the supportive community groups that had prayed for us. When those close to me fought uncontrollable tears, I comforted them.

One of those persons was Kathy Roberts, who wept profusely as she walked past me. The sixteen-year-old had made friends with John when he and her father (the man in the circular bed) were hospital roommates. Her mother had mentioned to me then that Kathy had a big crush on him.

Taking Kathy aside, I hugged her and said, "Don't cry for John, Kathy. Let him go. I talked with him just before he died, and he wanted to die. He probably is happier now than if he had lived." But I said this on blind faith. I had no proof of it.

Although such comforting words could offer solace to those outside my family, the only way I could calm my children was by giving them aspirin. Jack and I could not help each other. We both sensed that we would collapse if we showed any sentiment toward each other. While we struggled to maintain our composure, we managed to get through our obligations at the funeral home.

The Funeral and a New Beginning

We stood as a family with the pallbearers in the vestibule of St. Mary's Church, waiting for the hearse to arrive. When it pulled up to the curb, the pallbearers walked slowly down the steps to meet it. They then carried the casket up the steps and through the front doors, and placed it on a cart in front of us.

Mr. Howland, the funeral director, lined us up for the procession. He positioned Christopher between Jack and me. We were to walk behind the pallbearers. Rob and Lynn, walking together, were to follow us. With the sun streaming through the stained glass windows of the church, we started down the aisle. But the procession came to an abrupt halt when Christopher suddenly screamed. Knowing that his brother was in that casket, he now realized, perhaps for the first time, that any hope for John's survival was gone. Numbed by our own pain, Jack and I had not prepared him for this moment.

Stooping down, we hugged and comforted him. Then, with each of us putting a supportive arm around him, we continued down the aisle. At the left front pew, Mr. Howland stood waiting to seat us. Realizing that Jack and I would not be seated together if Christopher remained between us, he shook his head disapprovingly. Firmly taking hold of my arm, he pulled me in front of Christopher so that I would sit next to Jack, followed by Christopher and Lynn. Rob took the aisle seat.

When I looked across the aisle and saw caregivers from St. Luke's occupying the first two and a half rows of pews, I felt comforted. At that time, it was not common practice for hospital staff to attend funerals. Father

Cyril, Marcia, and Jim, a male orderly who had attended John during the final stage of his illness, were all there.

***

The next morning, Sylvia and I sat drinking coffee on the barstools in my kitchen. Exhausted from the strain of the preceding three days, we were still in our bathrobes. My sister had flown up from Florida to attend the wake and the funeral. Around 9 a.m. the doorbell started ringing. My three friends who had supported me at the hospital—Betty, Marty, and Nancy—arrived to join us within minutes of one another.

The five of us remained in the kitchen, drinking coffee and discussing the events of recent days. Still wondering why God had turned a deaf ear to my pleadings, I asked the group to consider why things had turned out so badly. Why did a child so young have to die? All was quiet as each of us pondered the question. But no one offered an answer.

Then I thought of a familiar passage from the Old Testament, Ecclesiastes 3:1–3: "To everything there is a season, and a time for every purpose under heaven: a time to be born, and a time to die…." I ventured, "Perhaps it is written at the time we are born when we will die. Perhaps John was meant to die young." Revisionists were saying that the books of the Old Testament and the Gospels of the New Testament were nothing more than beautiful poetry. I had never really believed that, but now it was hard to know what to believe. I was confused.

Although it seemed as if only a short time had passed, Marty suddenly looked at the clock and gasped. It was already noon. She hurried out the door to meet her husband for lunch.

About 3 p.m., Betty and Nancy departed. Sylvia accompanied them to the door and then came back into the kitchen, where I still sat on a stool in the corner. Standing in front of me at the sink, she let her shoulders slump as she took in the view that extended miles out into the valley.

We began chatting again, and as I bent over to take another sip of coffee, she said suddenly, "You know, I can't talk anymore." I looked up and saw that her eyes were rolled up and her lips were pursed. It was an expression she had often used when someone was intruding on her space.

"Daddy and John are right here," she said, motioning with her right elbow to the space between us.

Somewhat shocked, I repeated quickly, "Daddy? You mean Dad?" Sylvia had always called our father "Daddy," but when I got older I called him "Dad."

"Mmm-hmm," she nodded. She looked out the window again and gazed into the distance.

"And they're very happy," she continued. I remained silent, watching her.

"Suddenly I don't think the things that I thought were important are important anymore," she went on. I assumed that she meant material things, such as well-furnished houses, splendid cars, and fashionable clothes, which had always been her top priority. But I said nothing.

"They're right here!" she insisted again, looking toward me.

Although I did not doubt that it was possible, I replied quietly, "I don't feel them."

"I can't tell you how I feel!" she continued, placing her left hand on her chest. "It's the nicest feeling. I wish I could feel like this the rest of my life! I can't explain it!"

"Emotional?" I asked.

"Yes," she agreed, nodding. "Emotional! It makes you feel as if you'd like to go with them!" She was silent again for a moment, as if she were listening to someone. Looking out the window, her eyes scanned the green trees on the hills and the fertile flatlands below.

"Everything's all right at home," she said, again putting her hand to her chest. "I mean *my* home." Then, motioning toward the distance, she added, "My family's all right." Dave had stayed behind in Florida with Pete and Joey.

After another brief silence, she suddenly nodded and looked at me. "Everything's going to be all right," she said, as if repeating what someone had told her.

"Hmm," I said, thinking aloud. "Isn't it strange how God lets you know the things He wants you to know."

"Yes," she nodded. "I guess He's making me tell you."

Deep in thought for a moment, she then relaxed her posture, and we began to converse on other subjects, as if nothing had happened.

Turning to leave the room, Sylvia said, "Well, you know, I ought to go get dressed."

"I know it. I ought to, too," I replied.

Then, impulsively, my sister pulled a kitchen stool over to the counter and sat facing me. "You know," she said, "I guess that's why I hated to leave Fairfield when we moved. I was so close to Father Mullen." Sylvia had recently moved from New Jersey to Florida. "You know," she continued, "I asked him why God let a good boy like John, who had never done anything to anybody, suffer like that." And he said, "Well, God didn't let his own son live."

I nodded. We chatted a bit longer.

Then Sylvia said again, "Well, I've got to go get dressed." She left the room and went upstairs.

But I now sat frozen, stunned. I reviewed in my mind what my sister had said, and as I began to comprehend it, I felt a great burden lifted from my shoulders.

A few days later, when Betty, Marty, and Nancy were unable to control their tears, I consoled them by repeating my conversation with Sylvia. They accepted it quietly. However, my sister and I did not mention it again for three years. Emotions still ran high between us, and fearing that discussing the matter with her might minimize it, I just held on to it as a kind of life raft. When we finally did discuss it, Sylvia spoke of it matter-of-factly, but in tones that suggested reverence.

***

I drove Sylvia to the airport the next morning. By the time I returned home, I knew that I could keep my silence no longer. Christopher's piercing scream at the funeral still tugged at my heart. I ran upstairs to his bedroom, and saw that he was awake. I sat beside him, looked into his eyes, and told him about the events of the previous day. Then, smiling, I whispered, "*Christopher, John is happy, and he is with Grandpa! He told me not to worry! Everything will be all right!*"

As Christopher pondered this revelation, his glazed eyes began to brighten, and I sensed that the same burden that had been lifted from my shoulders was now removed from his.

John's body, as we knew it, had died, but his spirit had moved on to a higher plane. He was still alive, but much happier. He could walk and see again. He was with loved ones and free from pain. We had lost him only temporarily. Someday we'd all be together again! With joy in my heart, I realized that God had not abandoned me. He had come through after all! Alleluia!

EPILOGUE

June 2001

Thirty years have passed since this story began to unfold. However, cancer continues to rank second only to heart disease as the leading cause of death in America.[13]

When writing this book, it was never my intention—nor is it now—to promote the grape diet as a viable cancer treatment that is still to be used today. My purpose was solely to narrate the events that occurred while it was administered to my son in order to ease his pain during the last stages of his dreadful disease.

In 1997, researchers published reports praising the cancer chemopreventive activity of the grape. They named resveratrol, a component of the grape, as a potent inhibitor of the cellular activities associated with the initiation, promotion, and progression of tumors. After conducting hundreds of tests to find anti-cancer compounds in foods that were widely available as well as nontoxic, they determined that the grape was the likeliest candidate, and that resveratrol merited further investigation.[14]

---

13 *World Almanac and Book of Facts 2000*, Mahwah, New Jersey: Primedia Reference Inc., p. 892.

14 M. Jang and others, "Cancer Chemopreventive Activity of Resveratrol, A Natural Product Derived from Grapes," *Science*, vol. 275, no. 5297, January 10, 1997, p. 218.

In his well-documented book,[15] Dr. Ralph W. Moss, an internationally acclaimed science writer reports: "Despite a few bright spots, the statistics on cancer incidence and mortality continue to be gloomy."

It is my hope that we are on the threshold of a long-awaited discovery to provide relief from this horrible disease and the incalculable human suffering it causes.

---

15 Ralph W. Moss, *1996 Update of The Cancer Industry: The Classic Exposé on the Cancer Establishment*, New York: Equinox Press, 1996, p. vii.

About the Author

Barbara Redmond was a freelance writer from 1968 to 1978. During that time, her work was published seven times in national magazines. She also wrote articles that appeared in local newspapers. Following the death of her son, she became a member of a regional health planning council funded by the National Cancer Institute. That council reviewed a number of options to improve cancer care and selected hospice as an approach to receive additional study.

As chairman of a hospice education committee, Ms. Redmond worked with the head of the education department at a local hospital and a community college professor who taught a course titled "Death and Dying." Following her presentations to the news media, hospital medical staffs, and service organizations, a hospice was founded in her area in 1978.

In 1979, Ms. Redmond taught a class called "How To Get Published" for a community college, and then worked as an assistant in a museum's publications department.

Following a year of retirement in 1994, Ms. Redmond spent the next five years writing this book. She is a resident of New York State. In addition to writing, she enjoys playing bridge, exercising, and visiting her three children and four grandchildren, who live in Pennsylvania, Connecticut, and Maryland.

APPENDIX

Author's Note: After I wrote the first draft of this story in 1995, I visited my brother and sister-in-law in California. While there, I noticed Bianca Leonardo's advertisement in the newspaper, wherein she offered to read or edit manuscripts for a fee. When I returned home, following a letter of inquiry, I sent her this entire manuscript to read. Within a week or two, she telephoned me. I was surprised when she identified herself as the publisher of the book How to Conquer Cancer Naturally. *We talked for about 1½ hours. I am pleased that she graciously accepted my invitation to write this Appendix.*

Bianca Leonardo, (author, publisher, and owner of Tree of Life Publications, Joshua Tree, California. Publisher of the book *How to Conquer Cancer Naturally*, by Dr. Johanna Brandt, 1989, 1996. The original edition, entitled *The Grape Cure*, was published in 1928.)

The greatest discovery in the field of health in this century has been, tragically, almost entirely overlooked. It is a most interesting story.

Johanna Brandt, living in South Africa, contracted cancer. She struggled with the disease for nine years. She would fast, the disease would wane, but then return, because she was eating the wrong foods, especially meat. She stumbled upon the grape as a blood cleanser, and finally, not returning to a harmful diet, was totally healed.

Dr. Brandt was not the kind of person who could selfishly keep her discovery and good fortune to herself. She felt convinced that America, rich and powerful, would welcome her discovery with open arms, and made the great sacrifice of leaving her country, her husband and young children, for the U.S.

Her plan was to share this natural therapy without charge, to all who had a need. At first, she was totally ignored. It was a crucifixion. She wrote in Chapter I of her book, *The Grape Cure*:

> *Those who have drunk deeply of the cup of homesickness will understand. But this was no ordinary homesickness. It was not merely a longing for home and loved ones, or a yearning for the slumbering, sunlit vastness of South Africa. It was a state of mental and spiritual anguish charged with the unfathomable suffering of all the ages. It was my utter helplessness.*
>
> *To hold the key to the solution to one of the greatest problems of life and to have it rejected, untried, as worthless—that is to pass through the dark night of the soul. To have a mockery of worldly splendors thrust upon one as a substitute for an ideal—that is the temptation in the wilderness. To offer the gift of deliverance from pain and disease—freely, without money and without price and to see it spurned—that is crucifixion—Calvary.*

In the foreword in Dr. Brandt's book, La Forrest Potter, M.D., attributed the success of the grape mono-diet to the proteids in the grape. He wrote, "Proteids constitute the protoplasmic base of the human cells. They are the great body builders. If they contain toxins (poisons) they become the body destroyers. Because most of our conventional foods, medicines and sera are contaminated by these poisons, science has for years been searching for non-toxic proteids which will not disturb the colloidal integrity of the cells of the body by osmosis. The grape proteid seems to be in line with this search."

More recently, in an article, "GRAPES: great for grown-ups and kids," published in *The New Woman*, August, 1995, John D. Folts, PhD., professor of medicine at the University of Wisconsin Medical School, is cited because of his search for the "link between wine and well-being as a way to explain the 'French paradox'—the fact that the French sustain only one-third as many heart attacks as Americans, yet consume four times as much butter. Their moderate enjoyment of red wine, studies show, unclogs their arteries and thereby reduces their risk of heart disease," the article continued.

Because of the documented ill effects of excessive alcohol consumption, however, Folts sought a way to get the benefits of red wine in nonalcoholic form and "discovered that ordinary purple grape juice contains some of the same heart-helping ingredient as red wine.

'It isn't the alcohol,' Folts said. 'It's the flavonoids.'" Flavonoids, the compounds that help keep blood platelets from clumping together and sticking to artery walls, occur naturally in organic grape skins, stems, and seeds, and are available today in tablet form.

Although science had done no research on flavonoids in 1928, and little was commonly known about proteids, in her book, *The Grape Cure*, Johanna Brandt cited many testimonials of cancer patients in her clinic who were cured by the grape diet after their doctors had given them up to die.

Printed in the United States
21028LVS00006B/346-357